AN OVERVIEW OF RECENT AND ONGOING CLINICAL TRIALS FOR BREAST CANCER

Third edition

by Martine J. Piccart and Aron Goldhirsch
on behalf of the Breast International Group
edited by Carolyn Straehle and prepared in
collaboration with Breast Cancer Online

The information contained in this book is also available on Breast Cancer Online
(www.bco.org) and is updated on a regular basis. Breast Cancer Online is published and
maintained by Greenwich Medical Media Ltd.

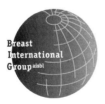

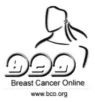

Breast Cancer Online
www.bco.org

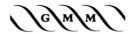

Greenwich Medical Media Ltd.
4th Floor, 137 Euston Road
London
NW1 2AA

ISBN 1-84110-205-9

First published 1996
2nd Edition 2000
3rd Edition 2003

Typeset by CharonTec Pvt. Ltd, Chennai, India

Printed by Ashford Colour Press, Gosport, UK

TABLE OF CONTENTS

FOREWORD 5

ACKNOWLEDGEMENT 6

LIST OF TOPICS 7

GROUPS, TRIALS UNITS AND RESEARCH PARTNERSHIPS CONTACT DETAILS 9

GROUPS, TRIALS UNITS AND RESEARCH PARTNERSHIPS STUDY DETAILS 59

ABCSG 61
ACCOG 73
AGO 81
ATLAS 87
BCIRG 91
BOOG 97
BREAST 103
DBCG 109
DRMAG 113
ECTO 115
EORTC 117
FNCLCC 131
GBG 135
GEICAM 153
GOIRC 169
GONO MIG 177
IBCSG 181
IBIS 199
ICCG 205
ICR-CTSU 217
IKA 227
JBCSG 233
NCIC CTG 235
NNBC-3 251
NWAST 255
PEGASE 259
SBG 263
WMBG 269
WSG 277
YBCRG 283

U.S. INTERGROUP 287

U.S. INTERGROUP CONTACT DETAILS 289
U.S. INTERGROUP STUDY DETAILS 297

FOREWORD

Several years have passed since the publication of the first edition of the BIG book on clinical trials for breast cancer, which grew out of the desire to give European clinical research in the adjuvant treatment of breast cancer an energetic push forward in terms of collaboration and efficiency. The book was seen as an instrument both to educate clinicians on the then current state of adjuvant clinical trials and to bring various research groups together, following the model of intergroup cooperation in North America. In the autumn of 1996, 23 representatives from collaborative groups in Europe and Canada – as well as one from the U.S. Intergroup – gathered in Bordeaux, and the Breast International Group – or BIG – was born. The first volume of the book was published shortly thereafter.

In 1999, BIG became an official international non-profit organization under Belgian law (aisbl), and its reach now expands well beyond its initial bounds: today's BIG consists of over 30 well-established, clinical research groups based in Europe, Australasia, Latin America and Canada, each with affiliated centers around the world. BIG's hope is that by bringing these organizations together to work towards answering critical questions in a short period of time – and with the necessary statistical power – research efficacy can be multiplied exponentially without compromising the identity of each member group.

A second edition of this book was published in mid-2000, followed now by a long awaited third edition. The spirit of the present volume remains the same as the first and second – to encourage care providers and investigators to consult what is available in clinical research for breast cancer. As in the past, it has welcomed contributions from BIG member groups as well as those who do not presently participate in our network. Some small changes have been introduced, however: To avoid duplication of trial information, where there have been multiple submissions of the same study, we have listed them under the name of the coordinating group only. Although they represent only a small number of studies in the book, some phase II, prevention, and metastatic breast cancer trials have been included at the request of contributors. We have also listed the contact information for several collaborative groups that are members of BIG, but that did not submit study information this time – or who may be participating in, rather than coordinating, one or more of the trials. Overall, the current edition contains 143 study summaries and the contact details for 45 groups, which is about double that of our very first edition.

The BIG book is accompanied by an internet version of the same, which allows contributors to update their entries at regular intervals and for new collaborative groups to be included as well. The electronic version of the book is hosted on Breast Cancer Online (www.bco.org), and was created and is maintained by Greenwich Medical Media in London (www.greenwich-medical.co.uk). But regardless of the medium, the purpose remains the same: to provide an essential educational resource and to lead to linkages and collaboration among academic research groups worldwide.

Martine J. Piccart, Aron Goldhirsch and Carolyn Straehle on behalf of the Breast International Group

Additional print copies of this book can be requested by contacting big@bordet.be.

ACKNOWLEDGEMENT

We would like to extend particular gratitude to all the groups who contributed their studies to this endeavor and to the clinical researchers and their teams whose diligence and dedication are the key to all progress in breast cancer research and benefit to patients and their families affected by the disease.

We are grateful to BIG's Pharmaceutical Industry Fund – specifically unrestricted educational grants from Amgen (Europe), AstraZeneca, Eli Lilly, F. Hoffmann La Roche, Schering Plough, Aventis and Bristol-Myers Squibb – for providing the financial resources necessary to publish the third edition and to support the development of an electronic counterpart on Breast Cancer Online.

LIST OF TOPICS

Anthracyclines 66–68, 70, 74, 75, 82, 94, 112, 116, 132, 142, 143, 146, 148, 151, 154, 155–158, 162, 167, 168, 172, 175, 178, 179, 206–208, 212, 224, 230, 231, 247, 252, 260, 261, 273, 278, 305, 306, 308, 309, 314
Aromatase inhibitors 63, 65, 69, 98, 200, 202, 249, 275, 312
Axilliary lymph node dissection 192, 300, 311
Bisphosphonates 69, 160, 166, 284, 313
Blood markers 310
Bone marrow micrometastasis 298
Bone mineral density 241, 284
Breast conservative treatment 127, 307
Cardiac function 310
Celecoxib 149, 214
DCIS 202, 307, 314, 317
Dose densification 82
Elderly patients 184
Fertility and chemotherapy 125
G-CSF secondary prophylaxis 76
Gemcitabine 162, 273
HER2 negative patients 92
HER2 positive patients 84, 94, 100, 107, 132, 303
High dose chemotherapy 67, 68, 74, 142, 143, 189, 209, 256, 260, 261, 264
Hormonal therapy 62, 63, 65, 66, 69, 98, 118, 136, 137, 139, 140, 142, 154, 164, 170, 182–186, 190, 194, 196, 197, 200, 202, 206, 208, 210, 218, 229, 230, 236, 238, 240, 241, 243, 249, 260, 261, 275, 302, 315,
Hormone receptor negative breast cancer 64, 67, 68, 140, 178
Hormone receptor positive breast cancer 71, 98, 110
Hormone replacement therapy 220, 267
Innovative schedules 170, 172, 187, 188
Locally advanced breast cancer 231
Loco-regional relapse 198
Low dose chemotherapy 191
Metastatic breast cancer 78, 100, 155, 157, 160, 161, 163–166, 303, 304, 306
Multiple drug resistance 114
Neutropenia 76
Node negative breast cancer 133, 136, 154, 156, 182, 183, 207, 228, 252
Node positive breast cancer 104, 110, 111, 112, 158, 179, 186, 188, 206, 208, 212, 230, 278, 280, 302, 308, 309
Ovarian suppression 110, 185, 194, 197, 218
Perioperative chemotherapy 64, 82, 84, 120, 124, 146, 148, 151, 168, 231
Postmenopausal patients 67, 71, 111, 139, 140, 183, 190, 200, 202, 206, 210, 212, 229, 230, 238, 275, 312, 314, 315
Predictive markers 129, 252
Premenopausal patients 62, 63, 65, 66, 67, 69, 98, 110, 112, 136, 137, 182, 185, 187, 194, 196, 197, 208, 218, 228, 236
Prevention 200, 202, 315

LIST OF TOPICS

Radiotherapy 122, 222, 245, 272, 317
Sentinel node micrometastasis 192, 298, 311
Serum lipids 243
Tamoxifen duration 88, 111, 229, 270
Taxanes 68, 70, 75, 78, 82, 84, 92, 94, 100, 104, 116, 129, 132, 146, 148, 151, 155–158, 162, 165, 167, 168, 179, 224, 234, 247, 252, 273, 278, 304–306, 308, 309
Trastuzumab 84, 94, 100, 107, 132, 165, 303, 306, 309
Treatment tailoring 256
Vinorelbine 161, 162
Young patients 125

GROUPS, TRIALS UNITS AND RESEARCH PARTNERSHIPS CONTACT DETAILS

Country: Austria

Group: Austrian Breast & Colorectal Cancer Study Group (ABCSG)

Chair: R. Jakesz
                    University of Vienna
                    Department of Surgery
                    Währinger Gürtel 18-20
                    A-1090 VIENNA
                    AUSTRIA
                    Tel: +43 1 404 00 6916
                    Fax: +43 1 404 00 6918
                    Email: Raimund.Jakesz@akh-wien.ac.at

Biostatistics Unit: M. Mittlböck
                    University of Vienna
                    Institute of Medical Computer Sciences
                    Währinger Gürtel 18-20
                    A-1090 VIENNA
                    AUSTRIA
                    Tel: +43 1 404 00 2276
                    Fax: +43 1 404 00 2278
                    Email: Martina.Mittlboeck@akh-wien.ac.at

Study Center: I. Mader
                    ABCSG Trial Center
                    Theresiengasse 32
                    A-1180 VIENNA
                    AUSTRIA
                    Tel: +43 1 4089230
                    Fax: +43 1 4090990
                    Email: Ines.Mader@akh-wien.ac.at

Country:	United Kingdom
Group:	Anglo-Celtic Cooperative Oncology Group **(ACCOG)**
Co-Chairs:	Prof R. Leonard South West Wales Cancer Institute Singleton Hospital Sketty Lane SWANSEA, SA2 8QA UNITED KINGDOM Tel: +44 1792 285 300 Fax: +44 1792 285 301
	Dr J. Crown St Vincent's Hospital Elm Park DUBLIN 4 IRELAND Tel: +353 1 269 50 33 Fax: +353 1 269 70 49
Administration Center:	Dr Liz Foster Scottish Cancer Therapy Network Trinity Park House South Trinity Road EDINBURGH, EH5 3SQ UNITED KINGDOM Tel: +44 131 551 8940 Fax: +44 131 552 4085

Country:	Germany
Group:	Associaton for Gynecologic Oncology (*Arbeitsgemeinschaft Gynäkologische Onkologie*) **(AGO)**
Chairman:	Prof Dr med Dr h.c.G. Bastert Universitätsfrauenklinik Voßstr. 9 69115 HEIDELBERG GERMANY Tel: +49 06221 567901
Vice Chairman:	Prof Dr R. Kreienberg Universitäts-Frauenklinik Prittwitzstr. 43 89075 ULM GERMANY Tel: +49 07031 502 7600
Chairman of AGO-subdivision breast:	PD Dr G. von Minckwitz Universitätsfrauenklinik Theodor-Stern-Kai 7 60596 FRANKFURT GERMANY Tel: +49 069 6301 7024
Website:	www.ago-online.de

Country:	Australia – New Zealand
Group:	Australian New Zealand Breast Cancer Trials Group **(ANZ BCTG)**
Group Coordinator and Director Operations Office:	Prof John F. Forbes ANZ Breast Cancer Trials Group Operations Office Dept of Surgical Oncology Newcastle Mater Misericordiae Hospital Locked Bag 7 HUNTER REGION MAIL CENTRE, NSW 2310 AUSTRALIA Tel: +61 2 4985 0113 Fax: +61 2 4960 1539 Email: john.forbes@anzbctg.newcastle.edu.au
Chair Scientific Advisory Committee:	Prof Alan Coates The Cancer Council Australia GPO Box 4708 SYDNEY, NSW 2001 AUSTRALIA Tel: +61 2 9036 3112 Fax: +61 2 9036 3111 Email: alancoates@cancer.org.au
Chair Board of Directors:	Dr Raymond Snyder Dept of Oncology St Vincent's Hospital Melbourne Healy Wing 41 Victoria Parade FITZROY, VIC 3065 AUSTRALIA Tel: +61 3 9288 3155 Fax: +61 3 9288 3172 Email: snyderrd@svhm.org.au
Group Statistician:	Prof John Simes ANZ BCTG Statistical Center NHMRC Clinical Trials Centre University of Sydney Locked Bag 77 CAMPERDOWN, NSW 2050 AUSTRALIA Tel: +61 2 9562 5002 Fax: +61 2 9565 1863 Email: john@ctc.usyd.edu.au

Head of Data Management:	Mrs Dianne Lindsay ANZ Breast Cancer Trials Group Operations Office Dept of Surgical Oncology Newcastle Mater Misericordiae Hospital Locked Bag 7 HUNTER REGION MAIL CENTRE, NSW 2310 AUSTRALIA Tel: +61 2 4985 0133 Fax: +61 2 4985 0141 Email: d.lindsay@anzbctg.newcastle.edu.au
Convenor Consumer Advisory Panel:	Assoc Prof Linda Reaby ANZ Breast Cancer Trials Group Senior Lecturer Faculty of Applied Science School of Nursing University of Canberra P.O. Box 1 BELCONNEN ACT 2616 AUSTRALIA Tel: +61 2 6201 2546 Fax: +61 2 6201 5128 Email: reaby@science.canberra.edu.au
Chair Prevention Studies Steering Committee:	Prof John F. Forbes ANZ Breast Cancer Trials Group Operations Office (see above)

Country:	International (Coordinating centre: UK)
Group:	Adjuvant Tamoxifen – Longer against Shorter **(ATLAS)**

Chair:
C. Williams
c/o CTSU
Radcliffe Infirmary
OXFORD, OX2 6HE
UNITED KINGDOM
Tel: +44 1865 4048 44
Fax: +44 1865 4048 45

Principal Investigator:
C. Davies
The ATLAS Trial Office
CTSU
Radcliffe Infirmary
OXFORD, OX2 6HE
UNITED KINGDOM
Tel: +44 1865 404 840
Fax: +44 1865 404 845
Email: christina.davies@ctsu.ox.ac.uk

International Advisor:
A. Goldhirsch
Oncology Institute of Southern Switzerland
Ospedale Civico
Via Tesserete 46
CH-6900 LUGANO
SWITZERLAND
Tel: +41 91 811 6515
Fax: +41 91 811 6517
Email: agoldhirsch@sakk.ch

ATLAS Trial Office:
CTSU
Radcliffe Infirmary
OXFORD, OX2 6HE
UNITED KINGDOM
Tel: +44 1865 404 844
Fax: +44 1865 404 845
Email: atlas@ctsu.ox.ac.uk

Country:	Argentina, Austria, Australia, Belgium, Brazil, Bulgaria, Bosnia, Canada, Colombia, Croatia, Czech Republic, Estonia, France, Germany, Greece, Hong Kong, Hungary, Ireland, Israel, Italy, Lebanon, Mexico, New Zealand, Poland, Portugal, Romania, Russia, Slovakia, Slovenia, South Africa, South Korea, Singapore, Spain , Sweden, Switzerland, Taiwan, United Kingdom, Uruguay, USA, Venezuela
Group:	Breast Cancer International Research Group **(BCIRG)**
Scientific Committee Chair:	Dennis Slamon, MD, PhD Chief, Division of Hematology / Oncology David Geffen School of Medicine at UCLA 10945 Le Conte Avenue, Suite 3360 LOS ANGELES, CA, 90095 Tel: +1 310 825 5193 Fax: +1 310 267 2301 Email: dslamon@mednet.ucla.edu
BCIRG Central Headquarters:	**Paris Office:** 13, rue Martin Bernard PARIS 75013 FRANCE Tel: +33 1 58 10 09 09 Fax: +33 1 58 10 08 77 Email address for all general inquiries and information: contact@cirg.org
BCIRG Satellite Offices:	**BCIRG Los Angeles Office:** 11111 Santa Monica Blvd., Suite 1750 LOS ANGELES, CA, 90025 USA Tel: +1 310 235 3445 Fax: +1 310 235 2662 **BCIRG Edmonton Office:** Suite 1100 9925-109 St. EDMONTON, ALBERTA T5K 2J8 CANADA Tel: +1 780 702 0200 Fax: +1 780 702 0190

Chief Medical Officer and Head of Clinical Research and Operations: Alessandro Riva, MD
13, rue Martin Bernard
PARIS 75013
FRANCE
Tel: +33 1 58 10 09 00
Fax: +33 1 58 10 09 12
Email: alessandro.riva@cirg.org

Director of Clinical Research: David Reese, MD
11111 Santa Monica Blvd., Suite 1750
LOS ANGELES, CA 90025
USA
Tel: +1 310 235 3451
Fax: +1 310 235 2662
Email: david.reese@cirg.org

Director of Scientific Development: Mary-Ann Lindsay, PharmD
Suite 1100
9925-109 St.
EDMONTON, ALBERTA T5K 2J8
CANADA
Tel: +1 780 702 0223
Fax: +1 780 702 0190
Email: mary-ann.lindsay@cirg.org

Statistician: Sandra Blitz, MSc
Suite 1100
9925-109 St.
EDMONTON, ALBERTA T5K 2J8
CANADA
Tel: +1 780 702 0200
Fax: +1 780 702 0190
Email: sandra.blitz@cirg.org

Director of Communications: Jim Mortimer, BA, HT
11111 Santa Monica Blvd., Suite 1750
LOS ANGELES, CA 90025
USA
Tel: +1 310 235 3483
Fax: +1 310 235 2662
Email: jim.mortimer@cirg.org

Website: www.bcirg.org

Country: The Netherlands

Group: Dutch Breast Cancer Trialist's Group **(BOOG)**

Chairman: Prof Dr J.G.M. Klijn
Erasmus MC/DDHK
P.O. Box 5201
3008 AE ROTTERDAM
THE NETHERLANDS
Tel: +31 10 4391733
Fax: +31 10 4391003
Email: j.g.m.klijn@erasmusmc.nl

Treasurer: Prof Dr J.W.R. Nortier
Leiden University Medical Center
Dept Clinical Oncology
P.O. Box 9600
2300 RC LEIDEN
THE NETHERLANDS
Tel: +31 71 5263057
Fax: +31 71 5266760
Email: j.w.r.nortier@lumc.nl

Secretary: Drs A.H. Westenberg
RADIAN, lok. Arnhem
Wagnerlaan 47
6815 AD ARNHEM
THE NETHERLANDS
Tel: +31 26 3712493
Fax: +31 26 4431200
Email: h.westenberg@radian.nl

Dr E.J.Th. Rutgers
Netherlands Cancer Institute/AvL
Plesmanlaan 121
1066 CX AMSTERDAM
THE NETHERLANDS
Tel: +31 20 5122551
Fax: +31 20 5122554
Email: e.rutgers@nki.nl

Office: Attn A.E. van Leeuwen-Stok, PhD
P.O. Box 9236
1006 AE AMSTERDAM
THE NETHERLANDS
Tel: +31 20 346 2547
Fax: +31 20 346 2525
Email: e.vanleeuwen@ikca.nl

Country:	Europe – Africa – South America – Middle East
Group:	Breast European Adjuvant Studies Team **(BREAST)**
Chair:	M.J. Piccart Jules Bordet Institute Chemotherapy Unit Rue Héger-Bordet 1 B-1000 BRUSSELS BELGIUM Tel: +32 2 541 3205 Fax: +32 2 538 0858 Email: martine.piccart@bordet.be
Data Center:	Jules Bordet Institute BREAST Operational Office Boulevard de Waterloo 121 B-1000 BRUSSELS BELGIUM Tel: +32 2 541 3181 Fax: +32 2 541 3090 Email: breast@bordet.be

Country: Central and Eastern Europe

Group: Central and East European Oncology Group **(CEEOG)**

Chair: J. Jassem
Medical University of Gdansk
Dept of Oncology and Radiotherapy
Debinki St., 7
PL-80211 GDANSK
POLAND
Tel: +48 58 520 38 99 – 349 22 70
Fax: +48 58 520 38 99 – 349 22 54
Email: jjassem@amg.gda.pl

Biostatistics Unit: A. Badzio, R. Dziadziouszko
Medical University of Gdansk
Dept of Oncology and Radiotherapy
Debinki St., 7
PL-80211 GDANSK
POLAND
Tel: +48 58 520 38 99 – 349 22 70
Fax: +48 58 520 38 99 – 349 22 54
Email: onkol@amg.gda.pl

Study Center: J. Laskowska
Medical University of Gdansk
Dept of Oncology and Radiotherapy
Debinki St., 7
PL-80211 GDANSK
POLAND
Tel: +48 58 520 38 99 – 349 22 70
Fax: +48 58 520 38 99 – 349 22 54
Email: onkol@amg.gda.pl

Country: Denmark

Group: Danish Breast Cancer Cooperative Group **(DBCG)**

Chair: P. Christiansen
Surgical Department
Aarhus Amtssygehus
2. Tage Hansensgade
8000 AARHUS C
DENMARK
Tel: +45 89 49 7508
Fax: +45 89 49 7549
Email: peer.christiansen@aas.auh.dk

DBCG Office: Rigshospitalet 7003
Blegdamsvej 9
2100 COPENHAGEN Ø
DENMARK
Tel: +45 35 38 65 30
Fax: +45 35 26 35 25
Email: dbcg@dgcg.dk

Country: Ireland

Group: Drug Resistance Marker Analysis Group **(DRMAG)**

Chair: Dr John Crown
                Consultant Medical Oncologist
                Medical Oncology Research Unit
                St Vincent's University Hospital
                Elm Park
                DUBLIN 4
                IRELAND
                Tel: +353 1 209 4839
                Fax: +353 1 283 7719
                Email: john.crown@icorg.ie

Study Center: Dr Lorraine O'Driscoll
                National Institute of Cellular Biotechnology (NICB)
                Dublin City University
                Glasnevin
                DUBLIN 9
                IRELAND
                Tel: +353 1 700 5700
                Fax: +353 1 700 5484
                Email: lorraine.odriscoll@dcu.ie

                Prof Martin Cynes
                National Institute for Cellular Biotechnology (NICB)
                Dublin City University
                Glasnevin
                DUBLIN 9
                IRELAND
                Tel: +353 1 700 5691
                Fax: +353 1 700 5484
                Email: martin.clynes@dcu.ie

Country:	Europe
Group:	European Cooperative Trial in Operable Breast Cancer **(ECTO)**
Chair:	L. Gianni Istituto Nazionale per lo Studio e la Cura dei Tumori Via Venezian 1 20133 MILAN ITALY Tel: +390 2 2390 2789 Fax: +390 2 2390 2678
Data Center:	Operations Office Istituto Nazionale per lo Studio e la Cura dei Tumori Via Venezian 1 20133 MILAN ITALY Tel: +390 2 2390 2206 / 2352 Fax: +390 2 2390 2678

Country:	Europe
Group:	European Organization for Research and Treatment of Cancer – Breast Cancer Group **(EORTC BCG)**
Chair:	Dr Emiel Rutgers The Netherlands Cancer Institute – Antoni Van Leeuwenhoekhuis Department of Surgery Plesmanlaan 121 NL-1066 CX AMSTERDAM THE NETHERLANDS Tel.: +31 20 512 2552 Fax: +31 20 512 2554 E-mail: erutgers@nki.nl
EORTC Data Center:	Avenue E. Mounier 83, bte 11 B-1200 BRUSSELS BELGIUM Tel: +32 2 774 16 11 Fax: +32 2 772 35 45
Website:	www.eortc.be

Country: France

Group: Fédération Nationale des Centres de Lutte contre le Cancer **(FNCLCC)**

Chair: H. Roché
Centre Claudius Regaud
20-24, rue du Pont St-Pierre
31052 TOULOUSE
FRANCE
Tel: +33 5 6142 4130
Fax: +33 5 6142 4624
Email: roche@icr.fnclcc.fr

Data Center: 101 rue De Tolbiac
75654 PARIS Cedex 13
FRANCE
Tel: +33 1 4423 0404

Country: Germany

Group: German Breast Group **(GBG)**

Chairs: Priv Doz Dr med Gunter von Minckwitz
             CEO, German Breast Group Forschungs GmbH
             C/o Klinikum der J.W. Goethe-Universität
             Klinik für Gynäkologie und Geburtshilfe
             Theodor-Stern-Kai 7
             60590 FRANKFURT
             GERMANY
             Tel: +49 69 6301 7024
             Fax: +49 69 6301 7938
             Email: minckwitz@em.uni-frankfurt.de

             M. Kaufmann
             J.W. Goethe Universität Frankfurt
             Dept of Obstetrics and Gynaecology
             Theodor-Stern-Kai 7
             D-60590 FRANKFURT
             GERMANY
             Tel: +49 69 6301 5115
             Fax: +49 69 6301 4717
             Email: kaufmann@em.uni-frankfurt.de

Data Center: I. Zuna / U. Räth
             Creative Research Solutions GmbH
             Wilhelmstr. 64
             D-65183 Wiesbaden
             GERMANY
             Tel: +49 611 97456 13
             Fax: +49 611 97456 66
             Email: ivan.zuna@creative-research-solutions.de

             M. Schumacher
             Institut für Medizinische Biometrie und Medizinische Informatik
             Universitätsklinikum Freiburg
             Stefan-Meierstr. 26
             D-76104 FREIBURG
             GERMANY
             Tel: +49 76 1203 6661
             Fax: +49 76 1203 6680
             Email: sec@imbi.uni-freiburg.de

Coordination: A.C. Diehl
German Breast Group
C/o J.W. Goethe Universität Frankfurt
Dept of Obstetrics and Gynaecology
Theodor Stern Kai 7
D-60590 FRANKFURT
GERMANY
Tel: +49 69 6301 7032
Fax: +49 69 6301 7310
Email: gabg@em.uni-frankfurt.de

Country: Brazil

Group: Grupo Brasileiro Cooperativo de Pesquisa em Oncologia Clínica (**GBOC**)

Chair: André Márcio Murad MD, PHD
Rua Piauí, 150
Sta. Efigênia
BELO HORIZONTE – MG – Brazil, 30.150-320
BRAZIL
Tel: +55 31 9984 3832 or 31 32413832
Fax: +55 31 32 41 3314
Email: murad@pib.com.br

Centers: José Bines, MD
Chief of Medical Oncology – INCA
Pça Cruz Vermelha, 238 and Centro
20.230-130 RIO DE JANEIRO – RJ Brazil
BRAZIL
Tel: +55 21 2506 6024
Fax: +55 21 2506 6025
Email: jbines@inca.gov.br

Carlos Gil Ferreira, MD, PHD
Rua Epitácio Pessoa, 4476/806 Bloco 1 Centro
22471-001 RIO DE JANEIRO – RJ Brazil
BRAZIL
Tel: +55 21 2506 6024
Fax: +55 21 2506 6025
Email: cferreira@inca.gov.br

Jefferson Vinholes
Rua Dna Laura, 226 s/202
Rio Branco
91430-090 PORTO ALEGRE – RS Brazil
BRAZIL
Tel: +55 51 3330 6031
Fax: +55 51 330 6031
Email: vinholes@santacasa.tche.br

André Moraes, MD
Av. dos Andradas, 2.287 sala 709
Sta. Efigênia
BELO HORIZONTE – MG – Brazil, 30.260-070
BRAZIL
Tel: +55 19 771 3798
Fax: +55 19 3289 1225
Email: amoraes@oncologia.com.br

Clarissa Matias, MD
Rua Clião Arouca, 115/12.002
40290-160 BROTAS - BA Brazil
BRAZIL
Tel: +55 71 331 8198
Fax: +55 71 245 9327
Email: mclarissa@yahoo.com

Country: Spain

Group: Grupo Español de Investigación en Cáncer de Mama **(GEICAM)**

Chair: M. Martín
Servicio de Oncología Médica
Hospital Universitario San Carlos
Ciudad Universitaria
28040 MADRID
SPAIN
Tel: +34 91 330 3546
Fax: +34 91 399 2627

Address: GEICAM (Spanish Breast Cancer Research Group)
Paseo de las Castellana 181, 16-Dcha
28046 MADRID
SPAIN
Tel: +34 91 4250620
Fax: +34 91 5710101
Email: geicam@geicam.org
Email2: geicam@geicamgroup.org

Website: www.geicam.org

Country:	Chile
Group:	Chilean Cooperative Group for Oncologic Research **(GOCCHI)**
Chairman:	Dr Jorge Gutiérrez GOCCHI Chilean Cooperative Group For Oncologic Research Avenida Américo Vespucio Norte 1314 Vitacura, SANTIAGO CHILE Tel: +56 2 208 9603 Fax: +56 2 207 6481 Email: jgutierr@clinicalascondes.cl
Vice-Chairman:	Dr Luis Orlandi Email: oncologia@csm.cl
Scientific Director:	Dr Rodrigo Arriagada Email: datacenter@gocchi.cl
Secretary:	Dr Eugenio Vinés Email: vines@iram.cl
Treasurer:	Dr Claudia Gamargo
Directors:	Dr Jorge Madrid Email: madrid@iram.cl Dr Waldo Ortuzar Email: wortuzar@ns.hospital.uchile.cl Dr Berta Cerda Email: bertacerda@hotmail.com Dr Nuvia Aliaga Email: naliagam@vtr.net Dr Alejandro Majlis Email: amajlis@entelchile.net Dr Octavio Peralta Email: octavioperalta@entelchile.net Dr Lucía Bronfman Email: luciabronfman@entelchile.net
Data Manager:	Mrs Maricarmen Zúñiga Email: maricarmen@gocchi.cl
Computer Programmer:	Mr Carlos Díaz Email: cdiaz@gocchi.cl
Secretary:	Mrs Carmen Paz Zepeda L. Email: datacenter@gocchi.cl

Country: Italy

Group: Italian Oncology Group for Clinical Research **(GOIRC)**

Chair: Prof Francesco Di Costanzo
                Unità Operativa di Oncologia Medica
                Azienda Ospedaliera Careggi
                Viale Pieraccini 17
                50139 Firenze
                ITALY
                Tel: +39 055 427 9648
                Fax: +39 055 427 7538
                Email: dicostanzofrancesco@tiscali.it;
                oncmed02@ao-careggi.toscana.it

Data Center: Dr.ssa Roberta Camisa, Dr.ssa Renata Todeschini
                Unità Operativa di Oncologia Medica
                Azienda Ospedaliera di Parma
                Via Gramsci 14
                43100 Parma
                ITALY
                Tel: +39 0521 702682
                Fax: +39 0521 995448
                Email: rcamisa@ao.pr.it; rtodeschini@ao.pr.it

Country:	Italy
Group:	Gruppo Oncologico Nord Ovest – Mammella Intergruppo (**GONO MIG**)
Chair:	Marco Merlano Azienda Ospedaliera S. Croce e Carle Via Michele Coppino 26 12100 Cuneo ITALY Tel: +390 171 441791 Fax: +390 171 441793 Email: merlano@sirio-oncology.it
Principal Investigator:	Lucia Del Mastro Istituto Nazionale per la Ricerca sul Cancro Largo R. Benzi 10 16132 Genova ITALY Tel: +390 10 5600 665 Fax: +390 10 5600 850 Email: lucia.delmastro@istge.it
Statistician and Data Center:	Paolo Bruzzi Servizio Sperimentazioni Cliniche Controllate Istituto Nazionale per la Ricerca sul Cancro Largo R. Benzi 10 16132 Genova ITALY Tel: +390 10 5737 477 Fax: +390 10 354103 Email: paolo.bruzzi@istge.it

Country: Greece

Group: Hellenic Breast Surgical Society (**HBSS**)
18-20 Tsoxa St.
11521 ATHENS
GREECE
Tel: +30 210 646 8180
Fax: +30 210 646 8218
Email: exem@hol.gr

Chair: Markopoulos Christos, MD, Mphil (UK), PhD
Associate Professor of Surgery – President of HBSS
Athens University Medical School
8 Iassiou St.
11521 ATHENS
GREECE
Tel: +30 210 722 1413
Fax: +30 210 724 7168
Email: cmarkop@hol.gr

Centers: Gogas Helen, MD, PhD
Lecturer in Medical Oncology
24 Karneadou St.
10675 ATHENS
GREECE
Tel: +30 6944 681 159 (mobile)
Fax: +30 210 778 1517
Email: hgogas@hol.gr

Dardoufas Konstantinos, MD, PhD
Associate Professor of Radiotherapy – Oncology
19 Filota St.
THRAKOMAKEDONES 13676
GREECE
Tel: +30 210 243 1091
Fax: +30 210 243 5013
Email: codar@hol.gr

Filippidis Theodoros, MD
Consultant Pathologist
18-20 Tsoxa St.
11521 ATHENS
GREECE
Tel: +30 210 643 6039

Gen. Secretary of HBSS:	Polychronis Athanassios, MD Consultant Surgeon 9 Ravine St. 11521 ATHENS GREECE Tel: +30 210 722 5577
Website:	http://www.exem.gr

Country:	Europe-America-Australia-Africa-Asia
Group:	International Breast Cancer Study Group **(IBCSG)**
Foundation Council Chair:	J. Collins Suite 16 Private Consulting Rooms Royal Melbourne Hospital Grattan St. PARKVILLE 3052 VICTORIA AUSTRALIA Tel: +61 9349 4688 Fax: +61 9347 3749 Email: collins@interspace.com.au
Scientific Committee Chair:	A. Goldhirsch Oncology Institute of Southern Switzerland Ospedale Regionale die Lugano (Civico) Via Tesserete 46 CH-6900 LUGANO SWITZERLAND Tel: +41 91 811 6515 Fax: +41 91 811 6517 Email: agoldhirsch@sakk.ch
	A. Coates Dept of Medical Oncology Royal Prince Alfred Hospital Missenden Road CAMPERDOWN, NSW 2050 AUSTRALIA Tel: +61 2951 57 680 Fax: +61 2951 91 546 Email: alancoates@cancer.org.com
Coordinating Center Studies Coordinator:	M. Castiglione IBCSG Coordinating Center Effingerstr. 40 CH-3008 BERN SWITZERLAND Tel: +41 31 389 9191 Fax: +41 31 389 9200 Email: monica.castiglione@ibcsg.org

Statistical and Data Management Center Director:	R.D. Gelber Dana-Farber Cancer Institute 44 Binney St. BOSTON, MA 02115 USA Tel: +1 617 632 3603 Fax: +1 617 632 2444 Email: gelber@jimmy.harvard.edu
Quality of Life Office Responsible Person:	Y. Wechsler IBCSG Coordinating Center Effingerstr. 40 CH-3008 BERN SWITZERLAND Tel: +41 31 389 9391 Fax: +41 31 389 9392 Email: yvonne.wechsler@ibcsg.org
Pathology Center Responsible Person:	B.A. Gusterson University of Glasgow Western Infirmary Royal Cancer Hospital The Haddow Hospital 15 Cotswold Road GLASGOW G11 6NT UNITED KINGDOM Tel: +44 141 211 2233 Fax: +44 141 337 2494 Email: bag57@clinmed.gla.ac.uk
	E. Viale European Institute of Oncology (EIO) Via Ripamonti 435 I-20141 MILANO ITALY Tel: +39 02 5748 9420 Fax: +39 02 5748 9417
Website:	www.ibcsg.org

Country: International

Group: International Breast Cancer Intervention Study Group **(IBIS)**

Co-Chairs: J. Cuzick
               Cancer Research UK Dept of Epidemiology
               Mathematics and Statistics
               Wolfson Institute of Preventive Medicine
               Charterhouse Square
               LONDON, EC1M 6BQ
               UNITED KINGDOM
               Tel: +44 207 882 6196
               Fax: +44 207 882 6252
               Email: jack.cuzick@cancer.org.uk

               J.F. Forbes
               Dept of Surgical Oncology
               University of Newcastle
               Newcastle Mater Misericordiae Hospital
               Locked bag 7
               HUNTER REGION MAIL CENTRE, NSW 2310
               AUSTRALIA
               Tel: +61 2 4921 1155
               Fax: +61 2 4929 1966
               Email: john.forbes@anzbctg.newcastle.edu.au

               A. Howell
               CRC Medical Oncology
               Christie Hospital
               Wilmslow Road
               WINTHINGTON
               MANCHESTER, M20 4BX
               UNITED KINGDOM
               Tel: +44 161 446 8037
               Fax: +44 161 446 8000 / 3299
               Email: maria.parker@christie-tr.nwest.nhs.uk

Trial office: Clare O'Neill
               IBIS, P.O. Box 123
               61, Lincoln's Inn Fields
               LONDON, WC2A 3PX
               UNITED KINGDOM
               Tel: +44 207 269 3151
               Fax: +44 207 269 3429
               Email: oneill@cancer.org.uk

Website: www.ibis-trials.org

Country:	Europe – Middle East – South America
Group:	International Collaborative Cancer Group **(ICCG)**
Chair:	P. Hupperets University Hospital Maastricht Internal Medicine Haematology / Oncology Postbus 5800 6202 AZ MAASTRICHT THE NETHERLANDS Tel: +31 (43) 387 7025 Fax: +31 (43) 387 5006 Email: phu@sint.azm.nl
Data Center:	ICCG Data Centre – Medical Oncology Division of Medicine Faculty of Medicine Imperial College London Charing Cross Campus LONDON, W6 8RF UNITED KINGDOM Tel: +44 (0)208 741 0648 Fax: +44 (0)208 741 0731 Email: iccg@imperial.ac.uk

Country: Ireland

Group: Irish Clinical Oncology Research Group (**ICORG**)

Chair: John Armstrong
Medical Board Office, St Luke's Hospital
Highfield Road
Rathagar, DUBLIN 6
EIRE
Tel: +353 (1) 497 4552
Fax: +353 (1) 497 2941
Email: john.armstrong@icorg.ie

Vice-Chair: John Kennedy
Dept of Haematology / Oncology, Hospital 1
St James's Hospital, James St.
DUBLIN 8
EIRE
Tel: +353 (1) 416 2169
Fax: +353 (1) 453 0557
Email: jkennedy@stjames.ie

Co-Chairs: John Crown
Breast Disease Specific Subgroup
Department of Medical Oncology
St Vincent's University Hospital
Elm Park, DUBLIN 4
EIRE
Tel: +353 (1) 209 4839
Fax: +353 (1) 283 7719
Email: john.crown@icorg.ie

Donal Hollywood
Radiation Modality Chair
Dept of Radiology, St Luke's Hospital
Highfield Road
Rathagar, DUBLIN 6
EIRE
Tel: +353 (1) 497 4552
Fax: +353 (1) 497 2941
Email: dhlywood@tcd.ie

Paul Redmond
Surgical Modality Chair
Dept of Surgery,
Cork University Hospital
COUNTY CORK
EIRE
Tel: +353 (21) 4920000
Fax: +353 (21) 4901240
Email: profredmond@eircom.net

Patrick Johnston
Medical Modality Chair
Dept of Oncology
Belfast City Hospital
51 Lisburn Road
BELFAST
UNITED KINGDOM
BT9 7AB
Tel: +44 (48) 90329241
Fax: +44 (48) 90263744

ICORG Central Office: Brian Moulton
Chief Executive Officer
120 Pembroke Road
DUBLIN 4
EIRE
Tel: +353 (1) 6677211
Fax: +353 (1) 6697869
Email: brian.moulton@icorg.ie

Tanya O'Shea
Project Manager – Breast
120 Pembroke Road
DUBLIN 4
EIRE
Email: Tanya.oshea@icorg.ie

Country:	United Kingdom
Trials Unit:	Institute of Cancer Research – Clinical Trials and Statistics Unit (ICR-CTSU)
Head:	J. Bliss Clinical Trials & Statistics Unit Section of Epidemiology The Institute of Cancer Research 15 Cotswold Road SUTTON SURREY, SM2 5NG UNITED KINGDOM Tel: +44 208 722 4297 Fax: +44 208 770 7876 Email: judith.bliss@icr.ac.uk
Deputy Head:	E. Hall Address as above Tel: +44 208 722 4292 Fax: +44 208 770 7876 Email: emma.hall@icr.ac.uk
Website:	www.icr.ac.uk/epidem

Country:	The Netherlands
Group:	Integraal Kanker Amsterdam **(IKA)**
Contact Person:	J. Benraadt, MD Deputy Director IKA Plesmanlaan 125 NL-1066 CX AMSTERDAM THE NETHERLANDS Tel: +31 20 346 2530 Fax: +31 20 346 2525
Data Center:	Plesmanlaan 125 NL-1066 CX AMSTERDAM THE NETHERLANDS Tel: +31 20 346 2544 Fax: +31 20 346 2525 Email: trialbureau@ikca.nl

Country: Italy

Group: Italian Trials in Medical Oncology (**ITMO**)

Chair: Prof Dr Emilio Bajetta
Istituto Nazionale per lo Studio e la Cura dei Tumori
Via Venezian 1
I-20133 MILAN
ITALY
Tel: +39 02 2390 2500
Fax: +39 02 2390 2149
Email: emilio.bajetta@istitutotumori.mi.it

Centers: Dr Nicoletta Zilembo
U.O. Oncologia Medica B
Istituto Nazionale per lo Studio e la Cura dei Tumori
Via Venezian 1
I-20133 MILAN
ITALY
Tel: +39 02 2390 4307
Fax: +39 02 2390 2149
Email: nicoletta.zilembo@istitutotumori.mi.it

Dr Roberto Buzzoni
Istituto Nazionale per lo Studio e la Cura dei Tumori
Via Venezian 1
I-20133 MILAN
ITALY
Tel: +39 02 2390 4307
Fax: +39 02 2390 2149
Email: roberto.buzzoni@istitutotumori.mi.it

Dr Luigi Celio
Istituto Nazionale per lo Studio e la Cura dei Tumori
Via Venezian 1
I-20133 MILAN
ITALY
Tel: +39 02 2390 2882
Fax: +39 02 2390 2149
Email: luigi.celio@istitutotumori.mi.it

Dr Giuseppe Procopio
Istituto Nazionale per lo Studio e la Cura dei Tumori
Via Venezian 1
I-20133 MILAN
ITALY
Tel: +39 02 2390 2557
Fax: +39 02 2390 2149
Email: giuseppe.procopio@istitutotumori.mi.it

Country: Japan

Group: Japan Breast Cancer Study Group **(JBCSG)**

Chair: Masakazu Toi MD
Tokyo Metropolitan Cancer and Infectious Disease Center, Komagome Hospital
3-18-22, Honkomagome
Bunkyo-ku
TOKYO 113-8677
JAPAN
Tel: +81 3 3823 2101
Email: maktoi77@wa2.so-net.ne.jp

Country: Mexico

Group: Mexican Oncology Study Group (**MOSG**)

Chair: Dr Laura Torrecillas Torres
MOSG
Parras 8-5
Hipodromo Condesa
MEXICO DF
Zip code 06100
MEXICO
Tel: +52 (55) 5258 5346
Fax: +52 (55) 5258 5490
Email: laura_torrecillas@prodigy.net.mx

Centers: Guadalupe Cervantes Sanchez, MD
Coyoacan 1344
Colonia del Valle
MEXICO DF
MEXICO
Tel: +52 (55) 5575 3072
Fax: +52 (55) 5575 3072
Email: gpecervantess@hotmail.com

Patricia Cortes Esteban, MD
Coyoacan 1344
Colonia del Valle
MEXICO DF
MEXICO
Tel: +52 (55) 5575 3072
Fax: +52 (55) 5575 3072
Email: patriciacortes@prodigy.net.mx

Country:	Canada
Group:	National Cancer Institute of Canada – Clinical Trials Group **(NCIC CTG)**
Chair:	K. Pritchard
	Toronto-Sunnybrook Regional Cancer Center
	2075 Bayview Avenue
	TORONTO, ONTARIO M4N 3M5
	CANADA
	Tel: +1 416 480 4616
	Fax: +1 416 480 6002
	Email: kathy.pritchard@tsrcc.on.ca
NCIC CTG Office:	Queen's University
	82-84 Barrie St.
	KINGSTON, ONTARIO K7L 3N6
	CANADA
	Tel: +1 613 533 6430
	Fax: +1 613 533 2941

Country:	United Kingdom
Group:	National Cancer Research Institute Breast Cancer Study Group **(NCRI)** (Partnership for government, charitable and private sectors)
BIG Voting Representative:	I. Smith Royal Marsden Hospital NHS Trust Dept of Medicine Downs Road SUTTON, SURREY SM2 5PT UNITED KINGDOM Tel: +44 208 661 3280 Fax: +44 208 643 0373 Email: Ian.Smith@rmh.nthames.nhs.uk
Group Address:	National Cancer Research Institute **(NCRI)** 20 Park Crescent LONDON W1B 1AL UNITED KINGDOM Tel: +44 207 670 5247 Fax: +44 207 670 5074 Email: info@ncri.org.uk
Website:	www.ncri.org.uk
Trials:	Please refer to those listed under UK collaborative groups or trials units

Country: Germany

Group: NNBC-3 Europe Trial Group **(NNBC-3)**
               Intergroup Study of AGO / WSG
               (in cooperation with EORTC RBG and BCG)

Chair: Prof Dr med Christoph Thomssen (PI)
               Prof Dr med Fritz Jaenicke
               Klinik und Poliklinik fuer Frauenheilkunde und Geburtshilfe
               Universitaetsklinikum Eppendorf
               University of Hamburg
               Martinistr. 52
               D-20246 HAMBURG
               GERMANY
               Tel: +49 40 42803 8172 / 3510
               Fax: +49 40 42803 2511
               Email: thomssen@uke.uni-hamburg.de, oben@uke.uni-hamburg.de

Coordinators: *Germany South*: PD Dr med Nadia Harbeck
               Frauenklinik und Poliklink der Technischen Universitaet Muenchen
               Klinikum rechts der Isar
               Ismaningerstr. 22
               D-81675 MUNICH
               GERMANY
               Tel: +49 89 4140 2437
               Fa: +49 89 4140 4846
               Email: nadia.harbeck@lrz.tu-muenchen.de

               Germany North: Dr med Volkmar Mueller
               Klinik und Poliklinik für Frauenheilkunde und Geburtshilfe
               Universitaetsklinikum Hamburg-Eppendorf
               Martinistr. 52
               D-20246 HAMBURG
               GERMANY
               Tel: +49 40 42803 8172 or 3510
               Fax: +49 40 42803 2511
               Email: vmueller@uke.uni-hamburg.de

               Europe: Prof Dr med Tanja Cufer
               Institute of Oncology
               Zaloška 2
               SI-1000 LJUBLJANA
               SLOVENIA
               Tel: +386 1 43 14 225
               Fax: +386 1 43 14 180
               Email: tcufer@onko-i.si

Laboratory Quality Assurance:

upA, PAI-1-determination:
Prof Dr CGJ Fred Sweep,
Experimental and Chemical Endocrinology
University Hospital Nijmegen
Katholieke Universiteit Nijmegen
Geert Grooteplein 8
NL-6500 HB NIJMEGEN
THE NETHERLANDS
Tel: +31 24 361 4279
Fax: +31 24 354 1484
Email: f.sweep@lev.azn.nl

HER-2/neu-determination:
Prof Dr med Josef Rüschoff
Institute for Pathology – Klinikum Kassel
Mönchebergstraße 41-43
D-34125 KASSEL
GERMANY
Tel: +49 561 980 – 3200 or 4001
Fax: +49 561 980 – 6983
Email: ruesch@klinikum-kassel.de

Statistician:

Prof Dr H.K. Selbmann, Christoph Meisner MA
IMI – Institut für Medizinische Informationsverarbeitung
Universität Tübingen
Westbahnhofstr. 55
D-72070 TÜBINGEN
GERMANY
Tel: +49 7071 29 85218
Fax: +49 7071 495 27
Email: christoph.meisner@med.uni-tuebingen.de

Country:	The Netherlands
Group:	Netherlands Working Party for Autotransplantation in Solid Tumors **(NWAST)**
Chair:	E.G.E. de Vries University Hospital Groningen Dept of Internal Medicine Division of Medical Oncology P.O. Box 30001 NL-9700 RB GRONINGEN THE NETHERLANDS Tel: +31 50 361 6161 Fax: +31 50 361 4862
Data Center:	The Netherlands Cancer Institute Dept of Biometrics Plesmanlaan 121 NL-1066 CX AMSTERDAM THE NETHERLANDS Tel: +31 20 512 2665 Fax: +31 20 512 2679

Country:	France
Group:	**PEGASE** Fédération Nationale des Centres de Lutte contre le Cancer (FNCLCC) et Société Française de Greffe de Moelle (SFGM)
Chair:	H. Roché Centre Claudius Regaud 20-24, rue du Pont St-Pierre 31052 TOULOUSE FRANCE Tel: +33 5 61 42 41 30 Fax: +33 5 61 42 46 24 Email: roche@icr.fnclcc.fr
Randomization:	Tel +33 1 45 83 93 94 or FNCLCC Fax: +33 1 45 84 66 82 Fax: +33 1 45 83 93 94

Country:	Scandinavian countries
Group:	Scandinavian Breast Group **(SBG)**
Chair:	J. Bergh Radiumhemmet Karolinska Institute & Hospital S-17176 STOCKHOLM SWEDEN Tel: +46 8 51 77 62 79 Fax: +46 8 51 77 51 96 Email: jonas.bergh@ks.se
Chair Clinical Trial Committee (CTC):	H.T. Mouridsen Dept of Oncology 5074 Rigshospitalet 9 Blegdamsvej 2100 COPENHAGEN Ø DENMARK Tel: +45 35 45 47 76 Fax: +45 35 45 69 66
CTC Office:	Rigshospitalet 9 Blegdamsvej 2100 COPENHAGEN Ø DENMARK Tel: +45 35 45 47 76 Fax: +45 35 45 69 66

Country: Peru

Group: Sociedad Peruana de Oncología Médica (**SPOM**)

Chair: Dr Carlos Vallejos Sologuren
Director Division de Medicina
Instituto de Enfermedades Neoplasicas
Angamos Este 2520
LIMA 34
PERU
Tel: +51 1 217 1300
Fax: +51 1 272 0309
Email: cvallejos@inen.sld.pe

Contact Person: Dr Henry Gomez
Director, Research Division
Instituto de Enfermedades Neoplasicas
"Dr Eduardo Caceres Graziani"
Av. Angamos Este 2520
LIMA 34
PERU
Tel: +51 1 217 1300
Fax: +51 1 271 1226
Email: gomezhenry@terra.com.pe

Country:	United Kingdom
Group:	West Midlands Breast Group **(WMBG)**
Chair:	Dr Christopher J. Poole Cancer Research UK Clinical Trials Unit Institute for Cancer Studies The University of Birmingham EDGBASTON BIRMINGHAM B17 2TT UNITED KINGDOM Tel: +44 121 414 3791 Fax: +44 121 414 3700 Email: poolecj@aol.com
Biostatistics Unit:	Ms Janet Dunn Cancer Research UK Clinical Trials Unit Institute for Cancer Studies The University of Birmingham EDGBASTON BIRMINGHAM B17 2TT UNITED KINGDOM Tel: +44 121 414 3791 Fax: +44 121 414 3700 Email: j.dunn@bham.ac.uk
Study Center:	Cancer Research UK Clinical Trials Unit Institute for Cancer Studies The University of Birmingham EDGBASTON BIRMINGHAM B17 2TT UNITED KINGDOM Tel: +44 121 414 3787 Fax: +44 121 414 3700

Country:	Germany
Group:	Westgerman Study Group **(WSG)**

Chair:

For AM03:
U. Nitz
Dept of Gynaecology
University of Düsseldorf
Moorenstraße 5
40221 DÜSSELDORF
GERMANY
Tel: +492118117550
Fax: +49211312283
Email: nitzu@uni-duesseldorf.de
www.brustcentrum.de

For AM02:
U. Nitz & W. Kuhn (AGO – Mamma)
Dept of Gynaecology
University of Bonn
Sigmund- Freudstr. 25
53105 BONN
GERMANY

Biostatistics Unit:

For AM02:
M. Scholz
Trium Analysis Online GmbH
C/o IMSE, TU München
Kilinikum r.d. Isar
Ismaninger Str. 22
81675 MÜNCHEN
GERMANY

For AM03:
K. Ulm
Klinikum rechts der Isar
Institut für Medizinische Statistik und Epidemiologie
Ismaningerstr. 22
81675 MÜNCHEN
GERMANY

Study Center:
Universitätsfrauenklinik Düsseldorf
Studienzentrale
Moorenstraße 5
40221 DÜSSELDORF
GERMANY

Country:	England
Group:	Yorkshire Breast Cancer Research Group **(YBCRG)**
Chair:	Mr M. Lansdown Consultant in General Surgery St James's University Hospital Beckett St. LEEDS LS9 7TF WEST YORKSHIRE ENGLAND Tel: +44 (0)113 206 4506 Fax: +44 (0)113 268 1340 Email: mark.lansdown@leedsth.nhs.uk
Biostatistics Unit:	Northern and Yorkshire Clinical Trials and Research Unit 17 Springfield Mount LEEDS LS2 9NG WEST YORKSHIRE ENGLAND Tel: +44 (0)113 343 1477 Fax: +44 (0)113 343 1471
Study Center:	Northern and Yorkshire Clinical Trials and Research Unit 17 Springfield Mount LEEDS LS2 9NG WEST YORKSHIRE ENGLAND Tel: +44 (0)113 343 1477 Fax: +44 (0)113 343 1471

GROUPS, TRIALS UNITS AND RESEARCH PARTNERSHIPS
STUDY DETAILS

ABCSG

STUDIES

ABCSG

Title: Adjuvant therapy with CMF vs goserelin plus tamoxifen in premenopausal, hormone-responsive, lymph node-positive or -negative patients. Study 5

Coordinator: R. Jakesz
University of Vienna
Department of Surgery
Währinger Gürtel 18-20
A-1090 VIENNA
AUSTRIA
Tel: +43 1 40400 6916
Fax: +43 1 40400 6918

Summary:
- Opened in December 1990
- Target accrual: 1050 patients

Objectives:

- To compare DFS and OS in patients treated with standard chemotherapy (cyclophosphamide + methotrexate + 5-fluorouracil) and patients treated with goserelin and tamoxifen;
- To compare toxicities.

Scheme:

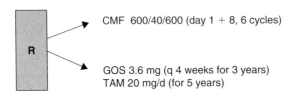

CMF 600/40/600 (day 1 + 8, 6 cycles)

R

GOS 3.6 mg (q 4 weeks for 3 years)
TAM 20 mg/d (for 5 years)

Update:

Study closed in June 1999 with 1034 patients.
Five-year results have been published (Jakesz et al, JCO 2002, 20: 4621–7).

Title: Adjuvant endocrine therapy in postmenopausal patients with hormone-responsive breast cancer: Tamoxifen vs tamoxifen plus aminoglutethimide. Study 6

Coordinator: R. Jakesz
University of Vienna
Department of Surgery
Währinger Gürtel 18-20
A-1090 VIENNA
AUSTRIA
Tel: +43 1 40400 6916
Fax: +43 1 40400 6918

Summary: • Opened in December 1990
• Target accrual: 2000

Study 6A: Rerandomization for recurrence-free patients in Study 6
Anastrozole 1 mg/d for 3 years vs control

Summary: • Opened in March 1996
• Target accrual: 812 patients

Objectives:

• To compare addition of aminoglutethimide to endocrine tamoxifen treatment with respect to OS, DFS and side effects (Study 6);
• After 5 years RFS, to compare anastrozole to control with respect to OS and DFS, to assess occurrence of second carcinoma (Study 6A).

Scheme:

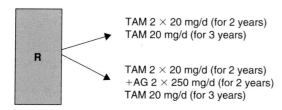

R

TAM 2 × 20 mg/d (for 2 years)
TAM 20 mg/d (for 3 years)

TAM 2 × 20 mg/d (for 2 years)
+AG 2 × 250 mg/d (for 2 years)
TAM 20 mg/d (for 3 years)

Update:

Study closed in December 1995 with 2021 patients, rerandomization completed in March 2001 with 812 patients. Five-year results have been published (Schmid et al, J Clin Oncol, 2003; 21: 984–90).

ABCSG

Title: Pre- and postoperative chemotherapy versus conventional adjuvant chemotherapy alone in patients presenting with hormone receptor-negative breast cancer.
Study 7

Coordinator: R. Jakesz
University of Vienna
Surgical Clinic
Department of General Surgery
Währinger Gürtel 18-20
A-1090 VIENNA
AUSTRIA
Tel: +43 1 404 00 6916
Fax: +43 1 404 00 6918

Summary:
- Opened in October 1991
- Target accrual: 480 patients

Objectives:

- To compare OS and RFS in patients treated with pre- and postoperative chemotherapy versus postoperative chemotherapy alone (cyclophosphamide + methotrexate + 5-fluorouracil and epirubicin + cyclophosphamide);
- To investigate to what percentage breast-conserving surgery may be enhanced by preoperative cytostatis.

Scheme:

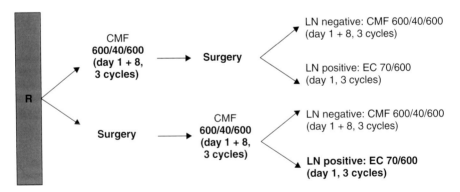

Update:

Study closed in October 1999 with 423 patients. Preliminary results have been published (Jakesz, Proc Am Soc Clin Oncol 2001, 20: 32a).

Title: Adjuvant endocrine therapy in postmenopausal patients with hormone-responsive breast cancer, G1 and G2 (ARNO). Study 8

Coordinator: R. Jakesz
University of Vienna
Department of Surgery
Währinger Gürtel 18-20
A-1090 VIENNA
AUSTRIA
Tel: +43 1 40400 6916
Fax: +43 1 40400 6918

Summary:
- Opened in January 1996
- Target accrual: 3500 patients

Objectives:

- To compare OS, RFS and side effects in postmenopausal patients with primary breast cancer, negative or positive nodes, and well or moderately differentiated tumors, treated with tamoxifen and then randomized to receive either tamoxifen or anastrozole;
- To additionally assess the value of adjuvant radiotherapy following breast-conserving surgery in lymph node-negative patients, T < 3 cm.

Scheme:

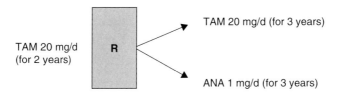

TAM 20 mg/d
(for 2 years)

R

TAM 20 mg/d (for 3 years)

ANA 1 mg/d (for 3 years)

Update:

3084 patients entered as of February 2003.

ABCSG

Title: Adjuvant chemotherapy in postmenopausal patients with hormone-responsive breast cancer, G3.
Study 9

Coordinator: R. Jakesz
University of Vienna
Department of Surgery
Währinger Gürtel 18-20
A-1090 VIENNA
AUSTRIA
Tel: +43 1 40400 6916
Fax: +43 1 40400 6918

Summary:
- Opened in January 1996
- Target accrual: 660 patients

Objective:

To compare OS, RFS and side effects in postmenopausal patients with primary breast cancer, negative or positive nodes, and undifferentiated, tumors, treated with adjuvant standard tamoxifen or additional epirubicin + cyclophosphamide.

Scheme:

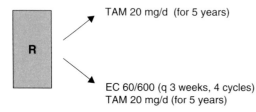

TAM 20 mg/d (for 5 years)

R

EC 60/600 (q 3 weeks, 4 cycles)
TAM 20 mg/d (for 5 years)

Update:

358 patients entered as of February 2003.

Title: Conventional vs high-dose combination chemotherapy in pre- and postmenopausal patients presenting with ⩾10 positive lymph nodes or ⩾4 positive lymph nodes and hormone receptor-negative disease. Study 10

Coordinator: R. Jakesz
University of Vienna
Department of Surgery
Währinger Gürtel 18-20
A-1090 VIENNA
AUSTRIA
Tel: +43 1 40400 6916
Fax: +43 1 40400 6918

Summary:
- Opened in July 1994
- Target accrual: 400 patients

Objective:

To compare RFS, OS, toxicity and quality of life in patients treated with 2 anthracycline-containing chemotherapy regimes (epirubicin + cyclophosphamide and cyclophosphamide + methotrexate + 5-fluorouracil), with different dosage intensities, in combination with tamoxifen, when indicated.

Risk factors:

>4 positive axillary lymph nodes or negative hormone receptor findings.

Scheme:

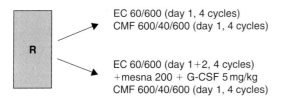

R → EC 60/600 (day 1, 4 cycles)
CMF 600/40/600 (day 1, 4 cycles)

R → EC 60/600 (day 1+2, 4 cycles)
+mesna 200 + G-CSF 5 mg/kg
CMF 600/40/600 (day 1, 4 cycles)

Update:

Study terminated in November 2001 with 112 patients.

ABCSG

Title: Adjuvant intensified conventional chemotherapy with epidoxorubicin + paclitaxel vs epidoxorubicin + paclitaxel and CTC with autologous peripheral stem cell transplantation in breast cancer patients at high risk for relapse.
Study 11

Coordinator: R. Jakesz
University of Vienna
Department of Surgery
Währinger Gürtel 18-20
A-1090 VIENNA
AUSTRIA
Tel: +43 1 40400 6916
Fax: +43 1 40400 6918

Summary:
- Opened in November 1997
- Target accrual: 240 patients

Objectives:

- To compare OS, RFS, quality of life, toxicity and morbidity;
- To assess the feasibility of high-dose chemotherapy CTC (cyclophosphamide + thiotepa + carboplatin) with autologous PSCT (peripheral stem cell transplantation) as compared to intensified conventional chemotherapy (epidoxorubicin + paclitaxel).

Risk factors:

>4 positive axillary lymph nodes or negative hormone receptor findings.

Scheme:

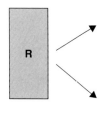

EPI + PAC 90/200 (q 3 weeks, 6 cycles)
+ G-CSF 5 mg/kg (from day 5)

EPI + PAC 90/200 (q 3 weeks, 3 cycles)
+ G-CSF 5 mg/kg (from day 5)
CTC 1500/125/200 (days -7 through -3)
+ mesna 1500 mg (days -7 through -3)
PSCT (day 0)

Update:

Study terminated in April 2002 with 108 patients.

Title: Adjuvant endocrine therapy and bisphosphonate therapy: Tamoxifen in comparison to anastrozole, alone or in combination with zoledronate, in premenopausal patients presenting with hormone-responsive, stage I and II breast cancer.
Study 12

Coordinator: R. Jakesz
University of Vienna
Department of Surgery
Währinger Gürtel 18-20
A-1090 VIENNA
AUSTRIA
Tel: +43 1 404 00 6916
Fax: +43 1 404 00 6918

Summary:
- Opened in June 1999
- Target accrual: 1250 patients

Objectives:

- To compare RFS and OS in patients treated with tamoxifen or anastrozole;
- To assess whether bisphosphonate treatment with zoledronate added to standard adjuvant therapy may improve RFS and OS.

Scheme:

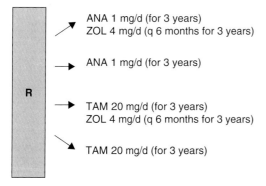

ANA 1 mg/d (for 3 years)
ZOL 4 mg/d (q 6 months for 3 years)

ANA 1 mg/d (for 3 years)

TAM 20 mg/d (for 3 years)
ZOL 4 mg/d (q 6 months for 3 years)

TAM 20 mg/d (for 3 years)

All patients receive basic therapy with GOS 3.6 mg (q 4 weeks for 3 years)

Update:

834 patients entered as of February 2003.

ABCSG

Title: Effect of 3 vs 6 cycles of epidoxorubicin/docetaxel + G-CSF upon the rate of complete pathological remissions in the neoadjuvant treatment of patients with primary breast cancer and no distant metastases.
Study 14

Coordinator: R. Jakesz
University of Vienna
Department of Surgery
Währinger Gürtel 18-20
A-1090 VIENNA
AUSTRIA
Tel: +43 1 40400 6916
Fax: +43 1 40400 6918

Summary:
• Opened in February 2001
• Target accrual: 282 patients

Objectives:

• To assess the rate of pathological complete remissions;
• To assess the rates of axillary lymph node metastases and breast-conserving procedures following 3 vs 6 cycles of epidoxorubicin (short infusion) / docetaxel (1-hour infusion).

Scheme:

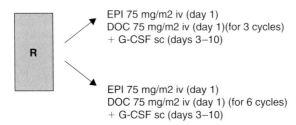

R

EPI 75 mg/m2 iv (day 1)
DOC 75 mg/m2 iv (day 1)(for 3 cycles)
+ G-CSF sc (days 3–10)

EPI 75 mg/m2 iv (day 1)
DOC 75 mg/m2 iv (day 1) (for 6 cycles)
+ G-CSF sc (days 3–10)

Update:

Study closed in December 2002 with 292 patients.

Title: Neoadjuvant hormonal therapy with exemestane in postmenopausal patients with primary hormone receptor-positive breast cancer and no distant metastases.
Study 17

Coordinator: R. Jakesz
University of Vienna
Department of Surgery
Währinger Gürtel 18-20
A-1090 VIENNA
AUSTRIA
Tel: +43 1 40400 6916
Fax: +43 1 40400 6918

Summary:
- Opened in September 2000
- Target accrual: 95 patients

Objective:

To evaluate efficacy in terms of clinical response (complete response, partial response, no change).

Scheme: Exemestane 25 mg/d (for 4 months)

Update:

79 patients entered as of February 2003.

ACCOG

STUDIES

ACCOG

Title: Intensive chemotherapy for high-risk (>4 axillary lymph nodes) breast cancer.
Study Anglo Celtic I

Coordinators: R. Leonard
South West Wales Cancer Institute
Singleton Hospital
Sketty Lane
SWANSEA
SA2 8QA
UNITED KINGDOM
Tel: +44 1792 285 300
Fax: +44 1792 285 301

J. Crown
St Vincent's Hospital
Elm Park
DUBLIN 4
IRELAND
Tel: +353 1 269 50 33
Fax: +353 1 269 70 49
Email: John.Crown@icorg.ie

Summary:
- Closed in June 1999 (opened in February 1995)
- Target accrual: 600 patients

Objective:

To determine the comparative efficacy of a high-dose sequential chemotherapy programme versus conventional CMF following doxorubicin induction in patients with high-risk primary breast cancer.

Scheme:

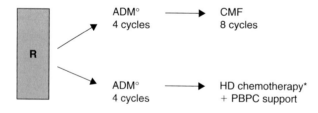

° ADM 75 mg/m^2 every 21 days
* cyclophosphamide 6.0 g/m^2 + thiotepa 800 mg/m^2

Update:

Study closed in June 1999.
605 patients entered.
Early results were presented by poster at ASCO 2002.

Title: Study Anglo Celtic II

Coordinator: J. Mansi
Oncology
St George's Hospital
Blackshaw Road
LONDON SW17 0Q
UNITED KINGDOM
Tel: +44 181 725 2955
Fax: +44 181 725 1199

J. Evans
Beatson Oncology Center
Western Infirmary
Dumbarton Road
GLASGOW G11 6NT
UNITED KINGDOM
Tel: +44 141 211 1741
Fax: +44 141 211 1830

Summary:
- Opened in October 1998
- Target accrual: 350 patients

Objective:

To compare the efficacy (response rates) and toxicity of Adriamycin and Taxotere versus Adriamycin and cyclophosphamide as primary medical therapy regimens in early breast cancer.

Scheme:

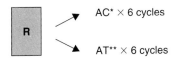

AC* × 6 cycles

AT** × 6 cycles

* AC   = Adriamycin 60 mg/m² plus
       cyclophosphamide 600 mg/m², iv q 3 weeks
** AT = Adriamycin 50 mg/m² plus
       Taxotere 75 mg/m², iv q 3 weeks

Update:

Study closed 2001.
363 patients entered.
Early results were presented by poster at ASCO 2002.

ACCOG

Title: Prospective randomized comparison of G-CSF (filgrastim) secondary prophylaxis vs conservative management of chemotherapy-induced neutropenia to maintain dose intensity in chemotherapy for breast cancer. Study Anglo Celtic III

Coordinator: Prof RCF Leonard
South Wales Cancer Institute
Singleton Hospital
Sketty Lane
SWANSEA
SA2 8QA
UNITED KINGDOM
Tel: +44 1792 285299
Fax: +44 1792 285301

Summary: Opened in October 2001
Target accrual: 816 patients

Objective:

To compare the effects of G-CSF secondary prophylaxis against standard management after the first neutropenic event in achieving planned dose intensity of chemotherapy for early breast cancer.

Scheme:

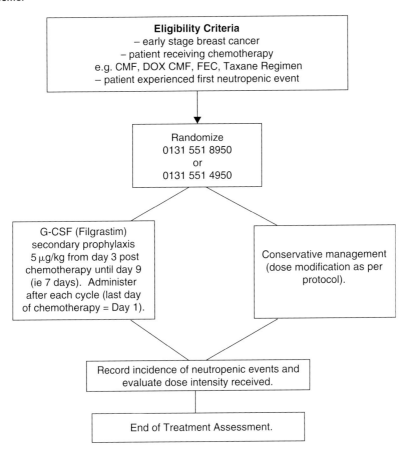

Eligibility Criteria
– early stage breast cancer
– patient receiving chemotherapy
e.g. CMF, DOX CMF, FEC, Taxane Regimen
– patient experienced first neutropenic event

Randomize
0131 551 8950
or
0131 551 4950

G-CSF (Filgrastim) secondary prophylaxis 5 μg/kg from day 3 post chemotherapy until day 9 (ie 7 days). Administer after each cycle (last day of chemotherapy = Day 1).

Conservative management (dose modification as per protocol).

Record incidence of neutropenic events and evaluate dose intensity received.

End of Treatment Assessment.

ACCOG

Title: A randomized 2-arm, prospective, multi-centre, openlabel phase III trial comparing the activity and safety of a weekly vs a 3 weekly paclitaxel treatment schedule in patients with advanced or metastatic breast cancer.
Study Anglo Celtic IV
"Will Weekly Win", www.taxol-uk.com

Principal Investigators: Dr Mark Verrill
Senior Lecturer in Medical Oncology
University of Newcastle Dept of Oncology
Newcastle General Hospital
Westgate Road
NEWCASTLE-UPON-TYNE, NE4 6BE
UNITED KINGDOM
Tel: +44 (0)191 219 4252
Fax: +44 (0)191 273 4867
Email: mark.verrill@ncl.ac.uk

Dr Dave Cameron
Western General Hospital
Edinburgh Cancer Centre
Crewe Road
EDINBURGH, EH4 XU
UNITED KINGDOM
Tel: +44 (0)131 537 2193
Fax: +44 (0)131 537 1029
Email: cameron@srv0.med.ed.ac.uk

Summary: Opened in September 2002
Target accrual: 600 patients

Objectives:

Primary:
- To compare the antitumour efficacy of weekly vs 3-weekly paclitaxel as determined by the time to disease progression;
- To study polymorphisms in the genes responsible for paclitaxel metabolism and link these to response rates and toxicity.

Secondary:
- To compare the toxicity of weekly vs 3-weekly paclitaxel;
- To compare the response rate of weekly vs 3-weekly paclitaxel;
- To compare overall survival in patients receiving weekly vs 3-weekly paclitaxel;
- To compare quality of life in patients receiving weekly vs 3-weekly paclitaxel.

Scheme:

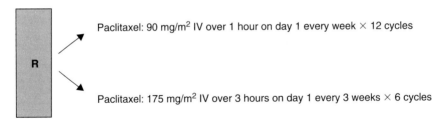

Paclitaxel: 90 mg/m^2 IV over 1 hour on day 1 every week $\times$ 12 cycles

Paclitaxel: 175 mg/m^2 IV over 3 hours on day 1 every 3 weeks $\times$ 6 cycles

Update:

Over 100 patients randomized to date (July 2003).

AGO

STUDIES

AGO

Title: Randomized controlled trial: Pre-operative, *dose-intensified, dose-dense,* sequential chemotherapy with epirubicin, paclitaxel and CMF $+/-$ darbepoetin a vs pre-operative, standard-dose, sequential chemotherapy with epirubicin and cyclophosphamide followed by paclitaxel $+/-$ darbepoetin $\alpha \times$ for breast cancer with T > 2 cm or inflammatory breast cancer. PREPARE – Pre-operative Epirubicin Paclitaxel Aranesp Study

Chair: PD Dr Michael Untch
Assistant Professor
Dept of Gynecology and Obstetrics
University of Munich
Klinikum Grosshadern
Marchioninistr. 15
D-81377 MUENCHEN
GERMANY
Tel: +49 89 7095 7581
Fax: +49 89 7095 7582
Email: muntch@helios.med.uni-muenchen.de
Website: www.ago-online.de

Summary:
- Phase III, multicenter study
- Opened June 2002
- Target accrual: 720 patients

Objectives:

- To evaluate the efficacy of dose-intensified, dose-dense preoperative chemotherapy with epirubicin, paclitaxel and CMF compared to standard-dose preoperative chemotherapy with epirubicin and cyclophosphamide, followed by paclitaxel, in patients with breast cancer ≥ 2 cm or inflammatory breast cancer;
- To evaluate the effect of additional administration of darbepoetin α in both therapy arms.

Primary end points:
- relapse free survival
- overall survival

Secondary end points:
- clinical remission rate
- histologic complete remission rate
- quality of life
- pathohistologic lymph node status
- correlation of clinical and histological remission rate with relapse free and overall survival

- peri-operative complications, evaluation of surgical margins after pre-operative chemotherapy, primary and secondary reexcisions to achieve free margins, rate of breast conservation and primary and secondary reconstructive procedures in both therapy arms

Scheme:

Arm A: Sequential therapy

Epirubicin 90 mg/m^2/Cyclophosphamide 600 mg/m^2, q21d × 4
Paclitaxel 175 mg/m^2, q21d × 4
±Darbepoetin alfa 1 × 4,5 µg/kg every 2 weeks

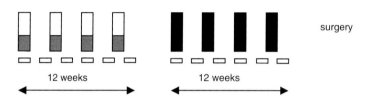

Arm B: Sequential, dose dense therapy

Epirubicin 150 mg/m^2, q14d × 3, G-CSF, 5 µg/kg/day, d3–d10
Paclitaxel 225 mg/m^2, q14d × 3, G-CSF, 5 µg/kg/day, d3–d10
CMF 500/40/600 mg/m^2, d1/d8, q28d × 3
±Darbepoetin alfa 1 × 4,5 µg/kg every 2 weeks

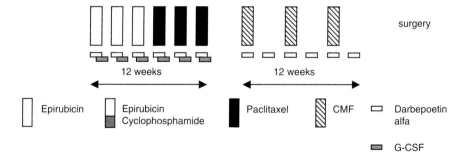

Update:

165 patients entered to date (July 2003).

83

AGO

Title: Preoperative chemotherapy with epirubicin / cyclophosphamide, followed by paclitaxel / trastuzumab, followed by post-operative therapy with trastuzumab for breast cancer with T > 2 cm or inflammatory breast cancer overexpressing HER2.
TECHNO Trial – *T*axol *E*pirubicin *C*yclophosphamide *H*erceptin *N*eoadjuvant

Chair: PD Dr Michael Untch
Assistant Professor
Dept of Gynecology and Obstetrics
University of Munich
Klinikum Grosshadern
Marchioninistr. 15
D-81377 MUENCHEN
GERMANY
Tel: +49 89 7095 7581
Fax: +49 89 7095 7582
Email: muntch@helios.med.uni-muenchen.de
Website: www.ago-online.de

Summary:
- Phase II, multicenter study
- Opened in June 2002
- Target accrual: 120 patients

Objective:

To evaluate efficacy and tolerability of sequential therapy with epirubicin / cyclophosphamide and a combination of paclitaxel / trastuzumab in the pre-operative treatment, followed by trastuzumab after surgery in patients with early breast cancer overexpressing Her2.

Primary end points:
- Safety: SAEs, cardial toxicity
- Efficacy: histologic remission rate at the time of surgery

Secondary end points:
- relapse-free and overall survival
- clinical and patho-histologic lymph node status
- clinical response rate
- correlation of clinical and histological remission rate with relapse free and overall survival
- peri-operative complications, evaluation of surgical margins after preoperative chemotherapy, primary and secondary reexcisions to achieve free margins, rate of breast conservation and primary and secondary reconstructive procedures
- quality of life by EORTC-questionnaire QLQ-C30

Scheme:

HER2/neu 3+ or 2+ (FISH pos.)

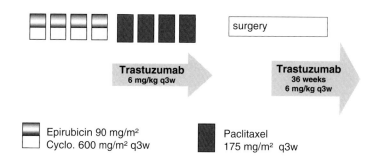

Update:

40 patients entered to date (July 2003).

ATLAS

STUDY

ATLAS

Title:	Phase III ATLAS Adjuvant Tamoxifen – Longer Against Shorter

Steering Committee Chair:
C. Williams
c/o CTSU
Radcliffe Infirmary
OXFORD, OX2 6HE
UNITED KINGDOM
Tel: +44 1865 404844
Fax: +44 1865 404845

Principal Investigator:
C. Davies
The ATLAS Trial Office
CTSU
Radcliffe Infirmary
OXFORD, OX2 6HE
UNITED KINGDOM
Tel: +44 1865 404 840
Fax: +44 1865 404 845
Email: christina.davies@ctsu.ox.ac.uk

International Advisor:
A. Goldhirsch
Oncology Institute of Southern Switzerland
Ospedale Civico
Via Tesserete 46
CH-6900 LUGANO
SWITZERLAND
Tel: +41 91 811 6515
Fax: +41 91 811 6517
Email: agoldhirsch@sakk.ch

Summary:

- Opened in June 1996
- Target accrual: 20 000 patients (fewer if survival benefit proved before)

Objective:

To assess reliably the balance of risks of prolonging the duration of adjuvant tamoxifen by at least 5 extra years among women who have already had about 5 years of tamoxifen and for whom there is uncertainty about whether they should stop now, or continue for longer.

Scheme:

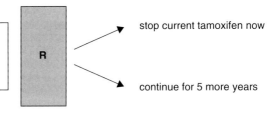

- breast cancer some time ago
- clinically free from disease
- currently on tamoxifen

R

stop current tamoxifen now

continue for 5 more years

Update:

11 200 patients entered to date (March 2003).

BCIRG

STUDIES

BCIRG

Title: A multicenter phase III randomized trial comparing docetaxel in combination with doxorubicin and cyclophosphamide (TAC) vs doxorubicin and cyclophosphamide followed by docetaxel (A → CT) as adjuvant treatment of operable breast cancer her2neu negative patients with positive axillary lymph nodes.
BCIRG 005

Chairs: Wolfgang EIERMANN, MD
Prof of Medicine
Medical Director
Red Cross Women Hospital
Fauenklinik vom Roten Kreuz, I Gyngebh. Abt./Taxisstr. 3
MUNCHEN 80637
GERMANY
Tel: +49 (89) 15 70 66 20
Fax: +49 (89) 15 70 66 23
Email: w.eiermann@gmx.net

John MACKEY, MD
Chair, Northern Alberta Breast Cancer Program
Cross Cancer Institute
11560 University Avenue
EDMONTON, ALBERTA, T6G 1Z2
CANADA
Tel: +1 (780) 432-8792
Fax: +1 (780) 432-8526
Email: johnmack@cancerboard.ab.ca

J. Crown
St Vincent Consulting Private Clinic
Herbert Avenue, Marian Road
DUBLIN 4
IRELAND
Tel: +353 1 209 4895
Fax: +353 1 283 7719
Email: john.crown@icorg.ie

Summary: • Start date: September 2000
• Target accrual: 3130 patients
• Enrollment completed: January 2003

Objectives:

Primary:
• Disease-free survival;

Secondary:
- Overall survival, toxicity and quality of life, pathologic and molecular markers, socioeconomics.

Scheme: *Patient Population:*

node-positive
adjuvant breast cancer
her2neu negative (centrally confirmed by FISH)

Randomization:

Stratify
- # of nodes (1–3, 4+)
- center

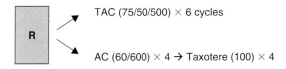

TAC (75/50/500) × 6 cycles

AC (60/600) × 4 → Taxotere (100) × 4

Update:

This study is complete for enrollment. The first interim analysis will be performed after the protocol specified number of events has been reached.

BCIRG

Title: Multicenter phase III randomized trial comparing doxorubicin and cyclophosphamide followed by docetaxel (AC → T) with doxorubicin and cyclophosphamide followed by docetaxel and trastuzumab (AC → TH) and with docetaxel, carboplatin and trastuzumab (TCH) in the adjuvant treatment of node positive and high risk node negative patients with operable breast cancer containing the HER2neu alteration.
BCIRG 006.

Chairs: D. Slamon
Chief, Division of Hematology / Oncology
David Geffen School of Medicine at UCLA
10945 Le Conte Avenue, Suite 3360
LOS ANGELES, CA 90095
USA
Tel: +1 (310) 825 5193
Fax: +1 (310) 267 2301
Email: dslamon@mednet.ucla.edu

J. Crown
St Vincent Consulting Private Clinic
Herbert Avenue, Marian Road
DUBLIN 4
IRELAND
Tel: +353 1 209 4895
Fax: +353 1 283 7719
Email: john.crown@icorg.ie

Dr Tadeusz Pienkowski
Memorial Cancer Centre – Institute of Oncology
Breast Cancer Clinic
5 Roentgena St.
02-781 WARSAW
POLAND
Tel: +48 (22) 644 0024
Fax: +48 (22) 644 0024
Email: tpien@coi.waw.pl

Summary:
- Enrollment Start date: April 2001
- Target Accrual: 3150 patients
- Planned interim cardiac analyses after 300, 900 and 1500 patients have received chemotherapy treatment and 6 months follow-up.

Objectives:

Primary:
- Disease-free survival;

Secondary:
- Overall survival, toxicity and quality of life, pathologic and molecular markers, socioeconomics.

Scheme: *Patient Population:*

node-positive, adjuvant breast or high-risk node-negative
her2neu positive (centrally confirmed by FISH in BCIRG laboratories)

Randomization:

Stratify
- # of nodes (0, 1–3, 4+)
- center

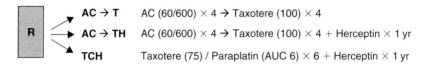

AC → T	AC (60/600) × 4 → Taxotere (100) × 4
AC → TH	AC (60/600) × 4 → Taxotere (100) × 4 + Herceptin × 1 yr
TCH	Taxotere (75) / Paraplatin (AUC 6) × 6 + Herceptin × 1 yr

Update:

Enrollment start: April 2001.
Expected enrolment completion: Early 2004.

BOOG

STUDIES

BOOG

Title: An open label randomized international multicenter comparative trial of 5 years adjuvant endocrine therapy with a LHRH agonist plus an aromatase inhibitor (Zoladex + Arimidex) vs 5 courses $FE_{90}C$ chemotherapy followed by the same endocrine therapy in pre or perimenopausal patients with hormone receptor-positive primary breast cancer.
BOOG 2002-01 / PROMISE

Principal Investigator: J.G.M. Klijn
Erasmus MC/DDHK
P.O. Box 5201
3008 AE ROTTERDAM
THE NETHERLANDS
Tel: +31 10 4391733
Fax: +31 10 4391003
Email: j.g.m.klijn@erasmusmc.nl

Summary: *Objectives:*

Primary:
Compare immediate optimal endocrine adjuvant therapy (Zoladex + Arimidex) with standard chemotherapy followed by the same optimal endocrine treatment in terms of time to recurrence of breast cancer (defined as the earliest local recurrence, new primary breast cancer, or death).

Secondary:
Measure overall survival.

Scheme: Hormonal treatment (Zoladex, Arimidex) will be given for 5 years or until confirmed 1st recurrence.

Chemotherapy (5 × FEC) will be given for 5 cycles.

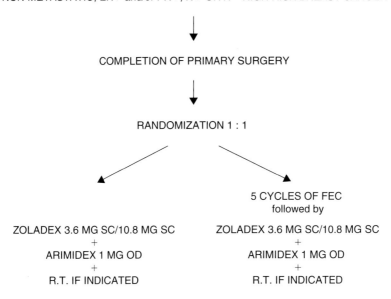

PRE-/PERIMENOPAUSAL WOMEN WITH INVASIVE
NON-METASTATIC, ER+ and/or PR+, N+ OR N− HIGH RISK BREAST CANCER

COMPLETION OF PRIMARY SURGERY

RANDOMIZATION 1 : 1

ZOLADEX 3.6 MG SC/10.8 MG SC
+
ARIMIDEX 1 MG OD
+
R.T. IF INDICATED

5 CYCLES OF FEC
followed by
ZOLADEX 3.6 MG SC/10.8 MG SC
+
ARIMIDEX 1 MG OD
+
R.T. IF INDICATED

Update:

Target accrual: Approximately 2300 patients.
Proposed start date: End 2003.

BOOG

Title: Open label, comparative, randomized, multicenter, study of trastuzumab (Herceptin®) given with docetaxel (Taxotere®) vs sequential single agent therapy with trastuzumab followed by docetaxel as first-line treatment for metastatic breast cancer (MBC) patients with HER2neu overexpression.
BOOG 2002-02 / HERTAX

Coordinators: Prof Dr J. Klijn, MD, PhD, Erasmus MC/DDHK, Rotterdam
Dr M. Bontenbal, MD, PhD, Erasmus MC/DDHK, Rotterdam
Dr C. Seynaeve, MD, PhD, Erasmus MC, DDHK, Rotterdam
P.O. Box 5201
3008 AE ROTTERDAM
THE NETHERLANDS
Tel: +31 10 4391733
Fax: +31 10 4391003
Email: j.g.m.klijn@erasmusmc.nl

Summary: *Indication:*

Patients with metastatic breast cancer with HER2*neu* overexpression (3^+ assessed by IHC DAKO HercepTest), previously untreated by chemotherapy, except for neoadjuvant or adjuvant (non-taxane containing) chemotherapy.

Primary endpoints:

Progression free survival, which is defined as follows:
• In the combination treatment arm: the time from start of treatment to progression or death, whichever occurs first;
• In the treatment arm with Herceptin (H) followed by Taxotere (TXT): the time from start of Herceptin treatment till progression during subsequent Taxotere treatment or death whichever occurs first;
• If a patient does not receive Taxotere once the patient progresses on or after Herceptin alone, for whatever reason, the time to progression is taken as the time to progression on or after Herceptin;
• If a patient goes off protocol treatment and receives off protocol any other hormonal treatment or chemotherapy without previous formal assessment of progression, the date of start of that other treatment is taken as the time of progression for the purpose of this study.

Secondary endpoints:

• Response rate. In the Herceptin followed by Taxotere arm, both the response on Herceptin and the response on Taxotere will be assessed;
• Overall survival measured from start of protocol treatment till date of death.

Target accrual: 100 patients (50 per arm)

Scheme: Comparative, randomized, multicenter, open-label, phase II study.

Update:

Started February 2003.

BOOG participation in International studies:
BOOG 2001-01 / TEAM trial
BOOG 2001-02 / AMAROS (EORTC 10981/22023)
BOOG 2002-04 / HERA (BIG 01-01 / EORTC 10011 / BO16348B)
BOOG 2003-01 (BIG 1-03, ICCG C/20/01, GABG 27)
BOOG 2003-02 (BIG 1-02 / IBCSG 27-02)

BREAST

STUDIES

BREAST

Title: An intergroup phase III trial to evaluate the activity of docetaxel, given either sequentially or in combination with doxorubicin, followed by CMF, in comparison to doxorubicin alone or in combination with cyclophosphamide, followed by CMF, in the adjuvant treatment of node-positive breast cancer patients.
BIG 02-98 / TAX 315

Chairs: M.J. Piccart
Jules Bordet Institute
Chemotherapy Unit
Rue Héger Bordet 1
B-1000 BRUSSELS
BELGIUM
Tel: +32 2 541 3205
Fax: +32 2 538 0858
Email: martine.piccart@bordet.be

J. Crown
St Vincent's Hospital
Elm Park
DUBLIN 4
IRELAND
Tel: +353 1 209 4895
Fax: +353 1 283 7719
Email: john.crown@icorg.ie

P. Francis
Peter MacCallum Cancer Institute
St Andrews Place
3002 EAST MELBOURNE (VIC)
AUSTRALIA
Tel: +61 3 9656 1700
Fax: +61 3 9656 1408
Email: pfrancis@petermac.unimelb.edu.au

Coordinator: A. Di Leo
Jules Bordet Institute
BREAST Operational Office
Rue Héger Bordet 1
B-1000 BRUSSELS
BELGIUM
Tel: +32 2 541 3180
Fax: +32 2 541 3090
Email: breast@bordet.be

Summary: • Opened in June 1998
• Target accrual: 2730 patients

Objectives:

Primary:
- To compare disease-free survival of an adjuvant treatment with doxorubicin followed by docetaxel, followed by CMF to doxorubicin followed by CMF in operable breast cancer patients with positive axillary lymph nodes;
- To compare disease-free survival of an adjuvant treatment with docetaxel in combination with doxorubicin followed by CMF to doxorubicin in combination with cyclophosphamide followed by CMF in operable breast cancer patients with positive axillary lymph nodes.

Secondary:
- To compare disease-free survival of an adjuvant treatment with docetaxel given either sequentially or in combination with doxorubicin and followed by CMF to doxorubicin alone or in combination with cyclophosphamide and followed by CMF in operable breast cancer patients with positive axillary lymph nodes;
- To compare disease-free survival of an adjuvant treatment with doxorubicin followed by docetaxel, followed by CMF to doxorubicin in combination with docetaxel followed by CMF in operable breast cancer patients with positive axillary lymph nodes (sequential mono-chemotherapy versus polychemotherapy);
- To compare overall survival of treatment arms;
- To compare toxicity of treatment arms;
- To evaluate pathologic and molecular markers for predicting efficacy;
- Socioeconomic data will be collected in order to be able to perform a socioeconomic analysis by country, when needed.

Scheme:

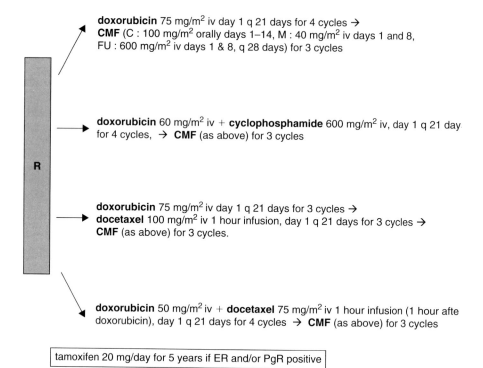

doxorubicin 75 mg/m² iv day 1 q 21 days for 4 cycles →
CMF (C : 100 mg/m² orally days 1–14, M : 40 mg/m² iv days 1 and 8,
FU : 600 mg/m² iv days 1 & 8, q 28 days) for 3 cycles

doxorubicin 60 mg/m² iv + **cyclophosphamide** 600 mg/m² iv, day 1 q 21 day
for 4 cycles, → **CMF** (as above) for 3 cycles

R

doxorubicin 75 mg/m² iv day 1 q 21 days for 3 cycles →
docetaxel 100 mg/m² iv 1 hour infusion, day 1 q 21 days for 3 cycles →
CMF (as above) for 3 cycles.

doxorubicin 50 mg/m² iv + **docetaxel** 75 mg/m² iv 1 hour infusion (1 hour afte
doxorubicin), day 1 q 21 days for 4 cycles → **CMF** (as above) for 3 cycles

tamoxifen 20 mg/day for 5 years if ER and/or PgR positive

Radiotherapy: Radiotherapy mandatory in case of breast-conservative surgery; allowed in
case of mastectomy, according to the policy in use at each participating center.

Update:

Trial closed 26 June 2001.
Total patients randomized is 2890.

Title:	HERA: A randomized three-arm multi-centre comparison of 1 year and 2 years of Herceptin® vs no Herceptin® in women with HER2-positive primary breast cancer who have completed adjuvant chemotherapy. BIG 01-01 / B016348

Chair: M. J. Piccart
Jules Bordet Institute
Chemotherapy Unit
Rue Héger-Bordet 1
B-1000 BRUSSELS
BELGIUM
Tel: +32 2 541 3205
Fax: +32 2 538 0858
Email: martine.piccart@bordet.be

Summary: *Objectives:*

Primary:
- To compare disease-free survival (DFS) in patients with HER2 overexpressing breast cancer who have been randomized to Herceptin® for one year versus no Herceptin®;
- To compare DFS in patients with HER2 overexpressing breast cancer who have been randomized to Herceptin® for two years versus no Herceptin®.

Secondary:
- To compare overall survival (OS) in patients randomized to i) Herceptin® for one year or no further therapy and to ii) Herceptin® for two years or no further therapy;
- To compare relapse-free survival (RFS);
- To compare distant disease-free survival (DDFS);
- To evaluate the safety and tolerability of Herceptin®;
- To compare the incidence of cardiac dysfunction in patients treated and not treated with Herceptin®;
- To compare outcomes (DFS, OS, RFS, DDFS, cardiac safety, overall safety) of patients treated with Herceptin® for one year compared with Herceptin® for two years.

Target accrual: 3192 patients

Scheme: Primary management pre HERA
(Surgery, [neo-]adjuvant chemotherapy + adjuvant radiotherapy)

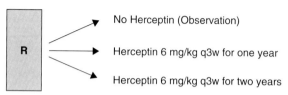

No Herceptin (Observation)

Herceptin 6 mg/kg q3w for one year

Herceptin 6 mg/kg q3w for two years

Update:

Trial opened in December 2001.
Accrual as of April 2003: 1360 patients.

DBCG

STUDIES

DBCG

Title   Adjuvant CMF vs castration in premenopausal receptor positive high-risk (node-positive or T > 5 cm) patients.
DBCG 89B

Chair: B. Ejlertsen
Dept of Oncology
Rigshospitalet
Blegdamsvej 9
2100 COPENHAGEN 0
DENMARK
Tel: +45 35 45 5088
Fax: +45 35 45 6966
Email: ejlertsen@rh.dk

Summary: • Closed in June 1998 (opened in January 1990)
• Target accrual: 750 patients

Objective:

To determine recurrence and mortality rate after primary surgery (and if necessary radiotherapy) supplemented by adjuvant therapy.

Scheme:

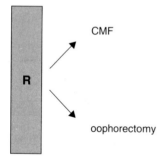

CMF

R

oophorectomy

Update:

Study closed in June 1998.
740 patients randomized.
960 patients not accepting randomization are also registered.
Reported at ASCO 1999.
Update ongoing.

Title: Adjuvant one year tamoxifen vs two years tamoxifen in post-menopausal receptor positive/unknown high-risk (node-positive or T > 5 cm) patients. DBCG 89C

Chair: J. Andersen
Dept of Oncology
Aarhus Komune Hospital
8000 AARHUS C
DENMARK
Tel: +45 86 12 5555
Fax: +45 86 13 9249

Summary: • Closed in January 1996 (opened in January 1990)
• Target accrual: 1000 patients

Objective:

To determine recurrence and mortality rate after primary surgery (and, if necessary, radiotherapy) supplemented by adjuvant therapy.

Scheme:

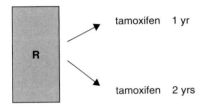

Update:

Study closed in January 1996.
2000 patients randomized.
541 patients not accepting randomization are also registered.
Update ongoing.

DBCG

Title: Adjuvant CMF vs CEF in high-risk (node-positive or T > 5 cm or premenopausal GII-III) patients.
DBCG 89D

Chair: HT Mouridsen
Dept of Oncology
Rigshospitalet
Blegdamsvej 9
2100 COPENHAGEN 0
DENMARK
Tel: +45 35 45 8500
Fax: +45 35 45 6966
Email: hmouridsen@rh.dk

Summary:
- Closed in June 1998 (opened in January 1990)
- Target accrual: 1500 patients

Objective:

To determine recurrence and mortality rate after primary surgery (and if necessary radiotherapy) supplemented by adjuvant therapy.

Scheme:

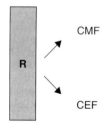

R

CMF

CEF

Update:

Study closed in June 1998.
1500 patients randomized.
1400 patients not accepting randomization are also registered.
Presented at ASCO 1999.
Update ongoing.

DRMAG

STUDY

DRMAG

Title: Drug Resistance Marker Analysis

Chairs: Dr John Crown
Medical Oncology Research Unit
St Vincent's University Hospital
Elm Park
DUBLIN 4
IRELAND
Tel: +353 1 209 2839
Fax: +353 1 283 7719
Email: john.crown@icorg.ie

Prof Martin Clynes
The National Institute for Cellular Biotechnology at Dublin
City University
Dublin City University
DUBLIN 9
IRELAND
Tel: +353 1 700 5691
Fax: +353 1 700 5484
Email: martin.clynes@dcu.ie

Summary: Cancers after initial shrinkage often regrow, and the cancer, is then resistant to the drugs used. Even worse, the regrowing cancer is also often cross-resistant to a range of other chemically and mechanically unrelated drugs. This phenomenon is known as multiple drug resistance (MDR).

Objective:

Attempts have been made to circumvent resistance by, for example, inhibiting drug efflux pumps, but to date no significant inroads have been made in treating MDR. More knowledge on mechanisms and definitions of new targets for therapeutic intervention is essential if this aspect of cancer is to be treated successfully, especially since MDR is recognised to be a multifactional phenomenon.
P-170 and MRP-1 analysis by IHC on paraffin embedded formalin fixed tissues. We also propose to analyse expression of specific cytochrome p540 enzymes, beclin-1, surviving and MDR3/Pgp-3

Scheme: Surgery / Biopsy
Tissue Fixation / Embedding
Section
Immunohistochemisty

ECTO

STUDY

ECTO

Title: European cooperative study of chemotherapy and surgery comparing adjuvant doxorubicin followed by CMF vs adjuvant doxorubicin / paclitaxel followed by CMF vs primary doxorubicin / paclitaxel followed by CMF in women with operable breast cancer and T > 2 cm.

Chair: L. Gianni
Istituto Nazionale per lo Studio e la Cura dei Tumori
Via Venezian 1
20133 MILANO, ITALY
Tel: +390 2 2390 206 / 352
Fax: +390 2 2390 678

Summary:
- Opened in November 1996
- Target accrual: 1250 patients

Objectives:

- To evaluate whether 8 cycles of primary chemotherapy before adequate surgery of breast tumor and loco-regional radiotherapy + tamoxifen for 5 years improves the disease-free (DFS) and overall survival (OS) in women with operable breast carcinoma and T > 2 cm in diameter at diagnosis;
- To assess whether, in the postoperative arms, the addition of paclitaxel to doxorubicin before CMF improves DFS and OS in these patients.

Scheme:

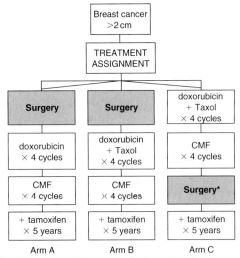

* whenever technically feasible: conservative surgery plus breast irradiation

Update:

Enrolment completed as of May 2002; 1355 patients.

EORTC

STUDIES

EORTC

Title: Postoperative adjuvant chemotherapy followed by adjuvant tamoxifen vs nil for node-negative and node-positive patients with operable breast cancer.
EORTC Study no. 10901

Coordinators: P.F. Bruning
Antoni van Leeuwenhoek Ziekenhuis
Plesmanlaan 121
NL-1066 CX AMSTERDAM
THE NETHERLANDS
Tel: +31 20 512 25 69
Fax: +31 20 512 25 72

R. Paridaens
Universitair Ziekenhuis Gasthuisberg
Afdeling Gezwelziekten
Herestraat 49
B-3000 LEUVEN
BELGIUM
Tel: +32 16 34 69 02
Fax: +32 16 34 69 01
Email: robert.paridaens@uz.kuleuven.ac.be

Summary:
- Closed in March 1999 (opened in March 1991)
- Target accrual: 1816 patients

Objectives:

- To investigate the disease-free interval and overall survival after adjuvant chemotherapy followed by tamoxifen compared to chemotherapy alone in patients curatively treated for primary breast cancer with surgery +/− radiotherapy;
- To investigate the influence of the estrogen receptor content of the primary tumor on the results of adjuvant treatment as given in this study.

Scheme:

POSTOPERATIVE ADJUVANT CHEMOTHERAPY*

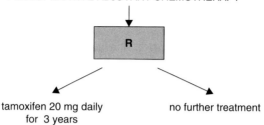

tamoxifen 20 mg daily   no further treatment
for 3 years

* CMF × 6 or FAC × 6 or FEC × 6 or CAF × 6 or CEF × 6 or AC × 4 or EC × 4

Update:

Study closed in March 1999.
1863 patients randomized.
Final analysis foreseen early 2004.
Evaluation in process.

EORTC

Title: Randomized phase III study comparing short, intensive preoperative combination chemotherapy with similar therapy given post-operatively. EORTC Trial 10902

Coordinators: M. Tubiana-Hulin
Centre René Huguenin
35 rue Daily
92211 SAINT-CLOUD Cedex
FRANCE
Tel: +33 1 471 11 515
Fax: +33 1 460 20 811

C.J.H. van de Velde
University Hospital
Dept of Surgery
P.O. Box 9600
NL-2300 RC LEIDEN
THE NETHERLANDS
Tel: +31 71 526 23 09
Fax: +31 71 526 67 50
Email: velde@surgery.azl.nl

J.P. Julien
Centre H. Becquerel
1 rue d'Amiens
76038 ROUEN Cedex
FRANCE
Tel: +33 2 32 08 22 12
Fax: +33 2 32 08 22 82

Summary:
- Closed in March 1999 (opened in March 1991)
- Target accrual: 550 patients (100/arm)

Objectives:

- To determine whether preoperative chemotherapy, by reducing the size of the primary tumor will permit more breast conserving therapies;
- To determine the disease-free interval and overall survival in patients who have received preoperative chemotherapy versus the same chemotherapy given postoperatively;
- To evaluate the response of the primary tumor to preoperative chemotherapy and correlate this response to disease-free and overall survival.

Scheme:

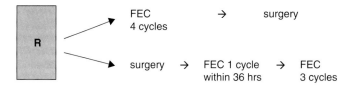

FEC = 600 mg/m^2 5-fluorouracil + 60 mg/m^2 Epirubicin + 600 mg/m^2 cyclophosphamide

Update:

The final results of the study have been published:
J.A. van der Hage, C.J.H. van de Velde, J.P. Julien, M. Tubiana-Hulin, C. Vandervelden, L. Duchateau, and Cooperating Investigators. Preoperative chemotherapy in primary operable breast cancer: Research and treatment of cancer trial 10902. J.Clin.Oncol.19, (Suppl.22): 4224-4237, 2001.

EORTC

Title: Phase III randomized trial investigating the role of internal mammary and medial supraclavicular (IM-MS) lymph node chain irradiation in stage I–III breast cancer (joint study of the EORTC Radiotherapy Cooperative Group and the EORTC Breast Cancer Cooperative Group). EORTC Study no. 10925 / 22922

Coordinators: W.F. van den Bogaert
Radiotherapy Department
U.Z. Gasthuisberg
Herestraat 49
B-3000 LEUVEN
BELGIUM
Tel: +32 16 346 917
Fax: +32 16 346 901

Dr H. Struikmans
Medisch Centrum Haaglanden – Westeinde
P.O. Box 432 – Lijnbaan 32
NL-2501 CK DEN HAAG
THE NETHERLANDS
Tel: +31 30 250 8800
Fax: +31 30 258 1226
Email: h.struikmans@mchaaglanden.nl

A. Fourquet
Institut Curie
Section Médecine et Hospitalière
Rue d' Ulm 26
75231 PARIS
FRANCE
Tel: +33 144 324 631
Fax: +33 144 324 616

H. Bartelink
Antoni van Leeuwenhoekhuis
Dept of Radiotherapy
Plesmanlaan 1121
NL-1066 CX AMSTERDAM
THE NETHERLANDS
Tel: +31 20 512 2122
Fax: +31 20 669 1101

Summary: • Opened in July 1996
• 4000 patients

Objectives:

To determine the effect of irradiation to the homolateral mammary suproclavicular lymph node chain in operable breast cancer on:
- overall survival
- disease-free survival
- metastases-free survival
- cause of death (breast cancer, cardiac, others).

Scheme:

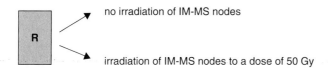

R → no irradiation of IM-MS nodes

R → irradiation of IM-MS nodes to a dose of 50 Gy

Update:

3744 patients randomized as of 1st July 2003.

EORTC

Title: Perioperative Endocrine Adjuvant Treatment (PEAT) – A double-blind Phase III clinical trial to compare the effects of a preoperatively administered single dose of "Faslodex" (long-acting ICI 182.780) with placebo on tumor recurrence in pre- and post-menopausal women treated for operable first primary breast cancer.
BIG 4-98 / EORTC Study no. 10963

Coordinators: C.J.H. van de Velde
University Hospital
Dept of Surgery
P.O. Box 9600
NL-2300 RC LEIDEN
THE NETHERLANDS
Tel: +31 71 526 23 09
Fax: +31 71 526 67 50
Email: velde@surgery.azl.nl

A. Howell
CRC Medical Oncology Christie Hospital
Wilmslow Road
MANCHESTER M20 4BX
WINTHINGTON
UNITED KINGDOM
Tel: +44 161 446 8037
Fax: +44 171 380 9920
Email: maria.parker@christie-tr.nwest.nhs.uk

Summary: • Open to accrual on the 30th of November 2000
• Closed to accrual on the 31st of October 2001

Objectives:

• To test the hypothesis that perioperative treatment with Faslodex may have an inhibitory effect on the development of metastasis, measured by disease-free survival and overall survival;
• To investigate possible toxicity.

Scheme:

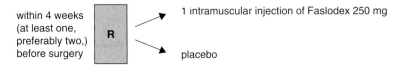

within 4 weeks (at least one, preferably two,) before surgery — **R** — 1 intramuscular injection of Faslodex 250 mg / placebo

Update:

Study closed due to low accrual on the 31st of October 2001.
Total patients randomized: 24.

Title: A survey of the Breast International Group (B.I.G.) to assess the attitude of patients aged less than 35 years, with early breast cancer, towards the risk of loss of fertility related to adjuvant therapies.
BIG 3-98 / EORTC 10002

Coordinator: A. DiLeo
Institut Jules Bordet
Chemotherapy Unit
1, rue Héger-Bordet
B-1000 BRUSSELS
BELGIUM
Tel: +32 2 541 3181
Fax: +32 2 541 3090
Email: angelo.dileo@bordet.be

Summary:
- Date of activation May 5th, 2003.
- Target accrual: 385

Objectives:

Primary endpoint:
- to estimate the attitude of breast cancer patients towards the risk of sterility related to anti-cancer treatments.

Secondary endpoint:
- to assess a possible relationship between patient attitude and (a) the fact that the patient already has children and (b) the time interval elapsed between the date of breast cancer diagnosis and the date of study participation.

Scheme: *Eligibility criteria:*

- female sex
- age < 35 years at time of breast cancer diagnosis
- previous or concomitant early breast cancer histologically / cytologically confirmed (stage I or II)
- no evidence of infertility
- no breast cancer relapse

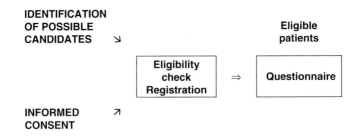

IDENTIFICATION OF POSSIBLE CANDIDATES ↘

Eligible patients

Eligibility check Registration ⇒ Questionnaire

INFORMED CONSENT ↗

Update:

11 patients randomized as of July 1st, 2003.

Title: LAMANOMA: Conservative local treatment vs mastectomy after induction chemotherapy in locally advanced breast cancer: a randomized phase III study.
BIG 2-00 / EORTC Study no. 10974-22002

Chair or Coordinator:
Pr. Jacek Jassem
Medical University of Gdansk
Dept of Radiotherapy
Ul. Debinki 7
PL-80 211 GDANSK
POLAND
Email: jjassem@amg.gda.pl

Dr Erik Van Limbergen
U.Z. Gasthuisberg
Dept of Radiotherapy
Herestraat 49
B-3000 LEUVEN
BELGIUM
Email: erik.vanlimbergen@uz.kuleuven.ac.be

Dr Geertjan van Tienhoven
Academisch Medisch Centrum
Dept of Radiotherapy
Meibergdreef 9
NL-1105 AZ AMSTERDAM
THE NETHERLANDS
Email: g.vantienhoven@amc.uva.nl

Summary:
- Open in October 2001
- Target sample size: 1300

Objectives:

- The main objective is to show that breast conservative treatment (BCT) (exclusive radiotherapy or tumorectomy followed or preceded by radiotherapy) is not inferior to mastectomy plus postoperative radiotherapy in terms of overall survival (primary endpoint) and time to locoregional failure (secondary endpoint) in locally advanced breast cancer patients who first received induction chemotherapy;
- Additionally, quality of life of the two strategies will be compared.

Scheme: *Stratification factors:*

- Institution
- Initial stage
- Response to induction chemotherapy
- Menopausal status

Eligible patients will be randomized between BCT (Breast Conservative Treatment) arm and Mastectomy Plus Radiotherapy arm

Update:

23 patients randomized as of July 1st, 2003.

Title:	p53 Study: First prospective intergroup translational research trial assessing the potential predictive value of p53 using a functional assay in yeast in patients with locally advanced / inflammatory or large operable breast cancer, prospectively randomized to a taxane versus non-taxane regimen. BIG 1-00 / EORTC 10994
Chair or Coordinator:	Dr Hervé Bonnefoi Hopital Cantonal Universitaire de Geneve Maternite Rue Micheli-du-Crest, 24 CH-1211 GENEVE 14 SWITZERLAND Email: herve.bonnefoi@hcuge.ch

Summary:
- Study open to accrual: March 2001
- Target sample size: 1440

Objectives:

- Compare two chemotherapy arms (arm A: without taxanes and arm B: with taxanes) in the two p53 subgroups separately;
- Test for an overall difference between the two chemotherapy arms;
- Test for interaction between the two chemotherapy arms and the p53 status.

Side studies:

- Agreement between p53 assessment by IHC method and functional test in yeast;
- Tumor assessment using cDNA Microarray technology.

Scheme:

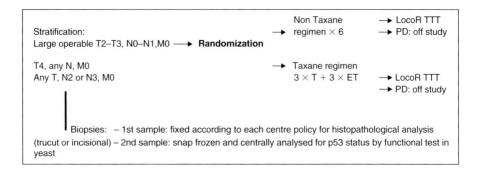

Update:

527 patients randomized as of July 1st, 2003.

FNCLCC

STUDIES

FNCLCC

Title: Randomized phase III trial comparing Docetaxel-Epirubicin to FEC for node positive non metastatic breast cancer patients. Randomization of Herceptin for HER2+++ patients.
PACS 04

Coordinator: Dr M. Spielmann
Institut Gustave Roussy
39, rue Camille Desmoulins
94 805 VILLEJUIF
FRANCE
Tel: +33 (0)1 42 11 43 35
Fax: +33 (0)1 42 11 52 31
Email: spielmann@igr.fr

Summary:
- Opened February 2001
- Target accrual: 2600 of whom 520 in the Herceptin part

Objectives:

- To compare disease free survival at 5 years after FEC or ET;
- A 10% increase of DFS at 3 years for patients receiving one year of Herceptin.

Scheme: N+, less than 65 y, unilateral breast cancer either 6 cycles of Epirubicin 75 mg/m^2, Taxotere 75 mg/m^2 or FEC 100 every 3 weeks.
Tamoxifen if ER or PR+.
For patients with hyperexpressing HER+++ tumors, second randomization after chemotherapy and radiotherapy between nothing or Herceptin every 3 week for one year.

Update:

1700 patients in January 2003.

Title: Randomized phase II trial comparing 4 to 6 cycles of FEC100 for node negative breast cancer patients.
PACS 05

Coordinator: Pr P. Kerbrat
Centre Eugène Marquis
Rue de la Bataille Flandres-Dunkerque
35 042 RENNES cedex
FRANCE
Tel: +33 (0)2 99 25 32 80
Fax: +33 (0)2 99 25 32 33

Summary: • Opened: September 2002
• Target accrual: 1512 women

Objective:

DFS at 5 years

Scheme: Node negative, more than 1 cm with at least one bad prognosis factor: $T > 2$ cm, ER and PR neg., grade II or III, age < 35 y.
4 or 6 cycles FEC100.
Tamoxifen if ER or PR+.

Update:

200 patients as of March 2003.

GBG

STUDIES

GBG

Title: Randomized trial with goserelin (2 years) vs CMF × 3 as adjuvant therapy of premenopausal breast cancer patients with node-negative and hormone receptor positive disease.
GABG-Study IV-A

Coordinator: Priv Doz Dr med Gunter von Minckwitz
CEO, German Breast Group Forschungs GmbH
C/o Klinikum der J.W. Goethe-Universität
Klinik für Gynäkologie und Geburtshilfe
Theodor-Stern-Kai 7
60590 FRANKFURT
GERMANY
Tel: +49 69 6301 7024
Fax: +49 69 6301 7938
Email: minckwitz@em.uni-frankfurt.de

Summary:
- Opened in November 1993
- Target accrual: 1400 patients

Objective:

To compare the use of a LH–RH analogue with a shortened (3 cycles) CMF-regimen in a lower risk group in terms of outcome and tolerability.

Scheme:

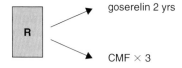

Update:

771 patients entered.
Trial closed February 2001.

Title: Randomized trial with postoperative, risk-adapted chemotherapy and a comparison of goserelin vs an observation group in premenopausal breast cancer patients.
GABG-Study IV-B

Coordinators: M. Kaufmann
J.W. Goethe Universität Frankfurt
Dept of Obstetrics and Gynaecology
Theodor Stern Kai 7
D-60590 FRANKFURT
GERMANY
Tel: +49 69 6301 5115
Fax: +49 69 6301 4717
Email: kaufmann@em.uni-frankfurt.de

W. Jonat
University of Kiel
Dept of Obstetrics and Gynaecology
Michaelisstr. 16
D-24105 KIEL
GERMANY
Tel: +49 431 597 2042 / 2040
Fax: +49 431 597 2149
Email: jonat@email.uni-kiel.de

Summary:
- Opened in November 1993
- Target accrual: 950 patients

Objective:

To compare the use of a LH–RH analogue with observation only after a risk-adapted sequential chemotherapy in terms of outcome and tolerability.

Scheme:

Study IV-B: node-negative or up to 3 positive nodes, receptor negative or 1–3 posititve nodes, receptor positive:

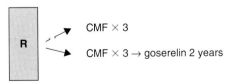

R
CMF × 3
CMF × 3 → goserelin 2 years

Study IV-B*: 4–9 positive nodes, receptor negative or positive:

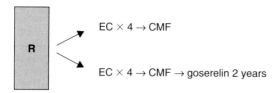

EC × 4 → CMF

EC × 4 → CMF → goserelin 2 years

Update:

Trial closed December 2000.
776 patients entered.

Title: Randomized trial with tamoxifen (5 years) vs tamoxifen (2 years) followed by anastrozole (Arimidex) (3 years) as adjuvant therapy of postmenopausal breast cancer patients with node-negative or node-positive (N 0–9) and hormone receptor positive disease and ≤ 75 years of age.
ARNO-Trial

Coordinators: W. Jonat
University of Kiel
Dept of Obstetrics and Gynaecology
Michaelisstr. 16
D-24105 KIEL
GERMANY
Tel: +49 431 597 2042 / 2040
Fax: +49 431 597 2149
Email: jonat@email.uni-kiel.de

M. Kaufmann
J.W. Goethe Universität Frankfurt
Dept of Obstetrics and Gynaecology
Theodor Stern Kai 7
D-60590 FRANKFURT
GERMANY
Tel: +49 69 6301 5115
Fax: +49 69 6301 4717
Email: kaufmann@em.uni-frankfurt.de

Summary:
- Closed in August 2002 (opened in 1996)
- Target accrual: 1000 patients

Objective:

To compare a single 5 years tamoxifen therapy with a sequential endocrine therapy (tamoxifen 2 years followed by anastrozole 3 years) in terms of outcome and tolerability.

Scheme:

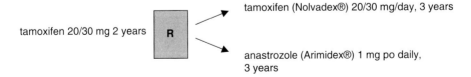

tamoxifen 20/30 mg 2 years → R →
tamoxifen (Nolvadex®) 20/30 mg/day, 3 years
anastrozole (Arimidex®) 1 mg po daily, 3 years

Update:

Study closed in August 2002.
1059 patients randomized.

GBG

Title: Randomized trial with postoperative, risk-adapted chemotherapy and a comparison between tamoxifen (5 years) and observation only in postmenopausal breast cancer patients with hormone receptor negative disease and ≤ 70 years of age.
GABG-Study IV-D

Coordinators: M. Kaufmann
J.W. Goethe Universität Frankfurt
Dept of Obstetrics and Gynaecology
Theodor Stern Kai 7
D-60590 FRANKFURT
GERMANY
Tel: +49 69 6301 5115
Fax: +49 69 6301 4717
Email: kaufmann@em.uni-frankfurt.de

W. Jonat
Universitätsklinikum Kiel
Dept of Obstetrics and Gynaecology
Michelisstr. 16
D-24105 KIEL
GERMANY
Tel: +49 431 597 2042 / 2040
Fax: +49 431 597 2146
Email:jonat@email.uni-kiel.de

Summary:
- Opened in November 1993
- Target accrual: 950 patients

Objective:

To compare a chemo-endocrine adjuvant therapy against chemotherapy alone.

Scheme:

Study IV-D: node-negative or up to 3 positive nodes:

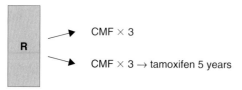

CMF × 3

CMF × 3 → tamoxifen 5 years

R

Study IV-D*: 4–9 positive nodes:

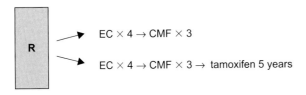

EC × 4 → CMF × 3

EC × 4 → CMF × 3 → tamoxifen 5 years

Update:

Study closed December 2000.
829 patients registered.

GBG

Title: Randomized trial with sequential EC / CMF chemotherapy vs high-dose Epirubicin chemotherapy simultaneously to a hormonal therapy depending on menopausal status in patients with 10 or more positive nodes and ≤ 70 years of age.
GABG-Study IV-E

Coordinator: W. Eiermann
Rotes Kreuz Krankenhaus
Dept of Obstetrics and Gynaecology
Taxisstr. 3
D-80637 MÜNCHEN
GERMANY
Tel: +49 89 15 70 66 20
Fax: +49 89 15 70 66 23
Email: wolfgang.eiermann@swmbrk.de

Summary:
- Opened in November 1993
- Target accrual: 460 patients

Objective:

To compare a sequential conventional dose chemotherapy against a high-dose monotherapy in high-risk patients.

Scheme:

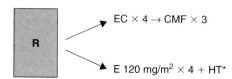

$EC \times 4 \rightarrow CMF \times 3$

$E\ 120\ mg/m^2 \times 4 + HT^*$

HT* = tamoxifen for postmenauposal women and goserelin for premenopausal women

Update:

Closed in December 2000.
Patients entered: 411.

Title: Adjuvant high-dose cyclophosphamide / thiotepa / mitoxantrone with autologous blood stem cell rescue for women with high-risk breast cancer. Prospectively randomized study of the GABG to compare 4 cycles Epirubicin / cyclophosphamide (EC) followed by high-dose cyclophosphamide / thiotepa / mitoxantrone (HD-CTM) with autologous blood stem cell rescue against 4 cycles Epirubicin / cyclophosphamide (EC) and 3 cycles cyclophosphamide / methotrexate / 5-fluorouracil (CMF) for women with high-risk breast cancer and ⩾ 10 histologically involved lymph nodes.
GBG-IV / EH-93

Coordinators: A.R. Zander / W. Krüger
Einrichtung für Knochenmarktransplantation
Medizinische Klinik
Universitätskrankenhaus Eppendorf
Martinistr. 52
D-20246 HAMBURG
GERMANY
Tel: +49 40 4717 4850 / 4851
Fax: +49 40 4717 3795

W. Jonat
Klinik für Gynäkologie und Geburtshilfe an der
Christian-Albrechts-Universität
Michaelistr. 16
D-24105 KIEL
GERMANY
Tel: +49 431 597 2042 / 2040
Fax: +49 431 597 2149
Email:jonat@email.uni-kiel.de

Prof. Alberti
Abteilung für Strahlentherapie und Radioonkologie
Radiologische Klinik
Universitätskrankenhaus Eppendorf
Martinistr. 52
D-20246 HAMBURG
GERMANY
Tel: +49 42803 6138
Fax: +49 42803 5192

D. Hossfeld
Medizinische Klinik
Hämatologie / Onkologie
Universitätskrankenhaus Eppendorf
Martinistr. 52
D-20246 HAMBURG
GERMANY
Tel: +49 42803 3962
Fax: +49 42803 8054

F. Jaenicke
Frauenklinik und Poliklinik
Universitätskrankenhaus Eppendorf
Martinistr. 52
D-20246 HAMBURG
GERMANY
Tel: +49 42803 2510
Fax: +49 42803 4355

M. Schumacher
Institut für Medizinische Biometrie und Medizinische Informatik
Abteilung Med. Biometrie und Statistik
Universitätsklinikum Freiburg
Stefan-Meier-str. 26
D-76104 FREIBURG
GERMANY
Tel: +49 761 203 6665
Fax: +49 761 203 6680
Email: bar@imbi.uni-freiburg.de

C. Schmoor
Institut für Medizinische Biometrie und Medizinische Informatik
Abteilung Med. Biometrie und Statistik
Universitätsklinikum Freiburg
Stefan-Meier-str. 26
D-76104 FREIBURG
GERMANY
Tel: +49 761 203 6665
Fax: +49 761 203 6680

Summary:
- Opened in November 1993
- Target accrual: 420 patients (90% power), 320 patients (80% power)

Objective:

To compare relapse free survival of women with high-risk breast cancer (pT0–3 or pT4B, pN1 ⩾ 10LN, M0) after adjuvant high-dose therapy (4* EC + HD − CTM + aPBSCT) with adjuvant standard therapy (4* EC + 3* CMF).

Scheme:

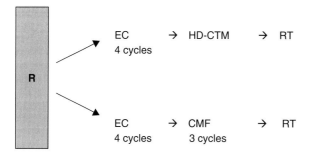

EC:	Epirubicin 90 mg/m², cyclophosphamide 600 mg/m², repeated every 21 days	
HD-CTM:	cyclophosphamide 1500 mg/m², thiotepa 150 mg/m², mitoxantrone 10 mg/m², given on days - 5 to - 2 prior to PBPC collection	
CMF:	cyclophosphamide 500 mg/m², methotrexate 40 mg/m², 5-fluorouracil 600 mg/m² (days 1 and 8), repeated every 21 days	
RT:	radiotherapy	

Update:

Study closed.
285 patients entered as of March 2003.

GBG

Title: A randomized, controlled, open phase II study comparing a combination of dose-intensified Adriamycin and Docetaxel with or without tamoxifen as preoperative therapy in patients with operable carcinoma of the breast (T $\geqslant$ 3 cm N0–2 M0).
GBG V study / GEPARDO

Coordinator: M. Kaufmann
J.W. Goethe Universität Frankfurt
Dept of Obstetrics and Gynaecology
Theodor-stern Kai 7
D-60590 FRANKFURT
GERMANY
Tel: + 49 69 6301 5115
Fax: + 49 69 6301 4717
Email: kaufmann@em.uni-frankfurt.de

Substudy Coordinators: S.D. Costa
J.W. Goethe Universität Frankfurt
Dept of Obstetrics and Gynaecology
Theodor-stern Kai 7
D-60590 FRANKFURT
GERMANY
Tel: +49 69 6301 4527
Fax: +49 69 6301 7034
Email: costa@em.uni-frankfurt.de

Priv Doz Dr med Gunter von Minckwitz
CEO, German Breast Group Forschungs GmbH
C/o Klinikum der J.W. Goethe-Universität
Klinik für Gynäkologie und Geburtshilfe
Theodor-Stern-Kai 7
60590 FRANKFURT
GERMANY
Tel: +49 69 6301 7024
Fax: +49 69 6301 7938
Email: minckwitz@em.uni-frankfurt.de

Summary:
- Closed in June 1999 (opened in April 1998)
- Target accrual: 200 patients

Objective:

To determine if the addition of tamoxifen to preoperative, dose-intensified Adriamycin and docetaxel combination chemotherapy can improve the rate of pathologically complete responses. The primary endpoint is defined as no microscopic evidence of viable tumour in the resected breast specimen.

Scheme:

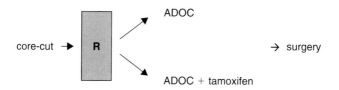

Update:

Study closed in June 1999.
250 patients randomized.

GBG

Title: A randomized, multicenter, open phase III study comparing a dose-intensified 8-week schedule of Adriamycin and docetaxel (ADOC) with a sequential 24-week schedule of Adriamycin / cyclophosphamide followed by docetaxel (AC-DOC) regimen as preoperative therapy in patients with operable carcinoma of the breast (T2–3 N0–2 M0).
GEPAR-DUO / GBG V

Principal Investigator: Priv Doz Dr med Gunter von Minckwitz
CEO, German Breast Group Forschungs GmbH
C/o Klinikum der J.W. Goethe-Universität
Klinik für Gynäkologie und Geburtshilfe
Theodor-Stern-Kai 7
60590 FRANKFURT
GERMANY
Tel: +49 69 6301 7024
Fax: +49 69 6301 7938
Email: minckwitz@em.uni-frankfurt.de

Summary:
- Opened in June 1999
- Target accrual: 1000 patients

Objective:

To determine whether the dose-intensified 8-week schedule of Adriamycin and docetaxel (ADOC) combination chemotherapy regimen is capable of obtaining a similar rate of pathologically complete responses as sequential 24-week schedule of Adriamycin / cyclophosphamide followed by docetaxel as a preoperative treatment for primary operable breast cancer. The primary end point is defined as no microscopic evidence of viable tumor (invasive and non-invasive) in all resected breast specimens and all axillary lymph nodes.

Scheme:

Measurable, operable, histologically confirmed breast cancer (T2–3, N0–2 M0)

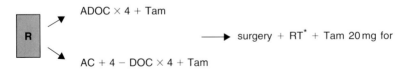

ADOC × 4 + Tam

AC + 4 − DOC × 4 + Tam

⟶ surgery + RT* + Tam 20 mg for

after breast conservation only
*in patients with pN+ disease further randomization in a subsequent protocol is recommended

Update:

Study closed.
913 patients entered as of June 2003.

Title:	A phase III multicentre double blind randomized trial of celecoxib vs placebo following chemotherapy in primary breast cancer patients BIG 1-03 – ICCG / C/20/01 – GBG 27 (see also description under ICCG)
Management:	Prof Charles Coombes, London (ICCG) Prof Bernd Gerber, München (GBG) Prof Pierre Hupperets, Amsterdam (ICCG) PD Dr Gunter von Minckwitz, Frankfurt (GBG) International Collaborative Cancer Group (ICCG) and the German Breast Group (GBG) intergroup study
Summary:	A multicentre, phase III, placebo controlled randomized trial. Patients are randomized between two years celecoxib and placebo in a 2:1 ratio in favour of celecoxib.

Chemotherapy:

Prior to randomization, all patients should have completed chemotherapy, preferably FEC75 3-weekly for 6 or 8 courses. However, other dose schedules of FEC plus combinations that contain EC followed by a taxane, or Epirubicin plus a taxane are permitted. CMF may be substituted for patients where Epirubicin is contraindicated, e.g. in cases where there is abnormal cardiac function.

Aims:

The primary aim is to assess the disease-free survival (DFS) benefit of two years adjuvant therapy with the COX-2 inhibitor celecoxib compared with placebo in primary breast cancer patients.

Secondary aims/endpoints:

- To compare overall survival;
- To define the safety of adjuvant therapy with celecoxib in this patient population;
- In HR positive patients, to compare tolerability of celecoxib with exemestane;
- To assess DFS benefit of two years adjuvant celecoxib compared with placebo in hormone receptor (HR) positive (i.e. ER positive and/or PR positive) and, if sufficient patients, HR negative (i.e. ER negative/PR negative) disease.

Scheme:

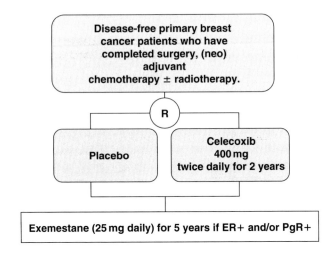

Update:

Planned study start: September 2003.

Title: A multi-center randomized phase II–III program evaluating 4 cycles of docetaxel, doxorubicin and cyclophosphamide (TAC) vs 4 cycles of vinorelbine and capecitabine (NX) as a salvage treatment in patients not sufficiently responding to 2 cycles of TAC and 4 cycles of TAC vs 6 cycles of TAC in patients sufficiently responding to 2 cycles of TAC as preoperative treatment of locally advanced (T4 a–d, N0–3,M0) or operable (T $\geq$ 2 cm, N0–2, M0) primary breast cancer. GEPAR-TRIO / GBG 12

Principal Investigator: Priv Doz Dr med Gunter von Minckwitz
CEO, German Breast Group Forschungs GmbH
C/o Klinikum der J.W. Goethe-Universität
Klinik für Gynäkologie und Geburtshilfe
Theodor-Stern-Kai 7
60590 FRANKFURT
GERMANY
Tel: +49 69 6301 7024
Fax: +49 69 6301 7938
Email: minckwitz@em.uni-frankfurt.de

Summary: *Design:*

Prospective, randomized phase III trial including an internal phase II trial
Phase II trial opened in September 2001
Phase III trial opened in July 2002

Study population:

Phase II trial: operable (T $\geq$ 2 cm, N0–2, M0) primary breast cancer (target accrual 2089 patients)
Phase III trial: locally advanced (T4 a–d, N0–3, M0) primary breast cancer (target accrual 170 patients)

Primary Objectives:

- To determine the pCR rate of 4 cycles of docetaxel, doxorubicin and cyclophosphamide (TAC) and of 4 cycles of vinorelbine and capecitabine (NX) (TAC vs NX) as a salvage treatment in patients not sufficiently responding (i.e. cNC) to 2 cycles of TAC as preoperative treatment of operable (T $\geq$ 2 cm, N0–2, M0) primary breast cancer;
- To determine the pCR rate of 6 cycles vs 8 cycles of docetaxel, doxorubicin and cyclophosphamide (TAC $\times$ 6 vs TAC $\times$ 8) in patients sufficiently responding (i.e. cPR or cCR) to the first 2 cycles of TAC as preoperative treatment of operable (T $\geq$ 2 cm, N0–2, M0) primary breast cancer.

Scheme:

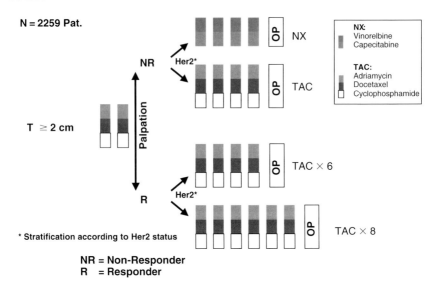

N = 2259 Pat.

NX:
Vinorelbine
Capecitabine

TAC:
Adriamycin
Docetaxel
Cyclophosphamide

NR

Her2*

NX

TAC

T ≥ 2 cm

Palpation

R

Her2*

TAC × 6

TAC × 8

* Stratification according to Her2 status

NR = Non-Responder
R = Responder

Update:

782 patients enrolled as of May 2003.

GEICAM

STUDIES

GEICAM

Title: Phase III study of concomitant vs sequential chemohormonotherapy (EC plus tamoxifen) as adjuvant chemotherapy for node-positive postmenopausal women.
GEICAM 9401

Coordinator: C. Picó
Servicio de Oncologia Médica
Hospital General de Alicante
Pza Dr Gómez Ulla, 15
03013 ALICANTE
SPAIN
Fax: +34 96 593 8448
Email: geicam@geicam.org

Summary:
- Opened in November 1994
- Closed in June 2001
- Results presented (oral presentation) at the 38th ASCO Annual Meeting (2002)

Objective:

To determine the best way to administer postsurgical chemotherapy plus tamoxifen (sequential vs concomitant) in node-positive postmenopausal breast cancer patients.

Scheme:

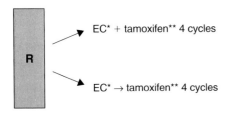

R
→ EC* + tamoxifen** 4 cycles
→ EC* → tamoxifen** 4 cycles

* EC: Epirubicin 75 mg/m^2 + cyclophosphamide 600 mg/m^2 day 1 every 3 weeks
** Tamoxifen: 20 mg/day for 5 years

Update:

Accrual completed in June 2001.
485 patients enrolled.
Final results were presented as oral communication at the 38th ASCO Annual Meeting (2002).

Title: A phase II trial for evaluation of sequential doxorubicin and docetaxel as first-line treatment in metastatic breast cancer.
GEICAM 9801

Coordinator: E. Alba
Servicio de Oncología Médica
Hospital U. Virgen de la Victoria
Colonia Santa Inés s/n
29010 MÁLAGA
SPAIN
Email: oncologia98@yahoo.com

Summary:
- Opened in April 1997
- Accrual completed in December 1999 with 81 patients

Objective:

To evaluate the efficacy and the toxicity profile of the sequential administration of doxorubicin and docetaxel as first-line chemotherapy in metastatic breast cancer.

Scheme: Doxorubicin 75 mg/m2 day 1 every 3 weeks (3 courses) followed by docetaxel 100 mg/m2 day 1 every 3 weeks (3 courses).

Update:

Results published in Breast Cancer Research and Treatment 77: 1–8, 2003.

GEICAM

Title: A multicenter phase III randomized trial comparing docetaxel with doxorubicin and cyclophosphamide (TAC) vs 5-fluorouracil with doxorubicin and cyclophosphamide (FAC) as adjuvant treatment of operable breast cancer patients with negative axillary lymph nodes. TARGET 0 / GEICAM 9805

Coordinators: M. Martin
Servicio de Oncología Médica
Hospital Clínico San Carlos
MADRID, SPAIN
Email: martín@geicam.org

A. Barnadas
Servicio de Oncología Médica
Hospital Germans Trias i Pujol
BADALONA- BARCELONA, SPAIN
Email: barnadas@ns.hugtip.scs.es

A. Lluch
Servicio de Oncología Médica
Hospital Clínico Universitario
VALENCIA, SPAIN
Email: ana.lluch@uv.es

Summary:
- Opened in June 1999
- Target accrual: 1054 patients

Objective:

To determine the relative efficacy and toxicity of docetaxel in combination with doxorubicin and cyclophosphomide (TAC) vs 5-fluorouracil in combination with doxorubicin and cyclophosphamide (FAC) as adjuvant chemotherapy for high-risk (St Gallen criteria) node-negative breast cancer.

Scheme:

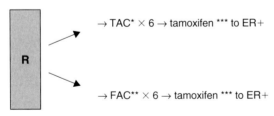

$\rightarrow$ TAC* $\times$ 6 $\rightarrow$ tamoxifen *** to ER+

R

$\rightarrow$ FAC** $\times$ 6 $\rightarrow$ tamoxifen *** to ER+

* Taxotere 75 mg/m^2 + Doxorubicin 50 mg/m^2 day + cyclophosphamide 500 mg/ m^2, day 1 every 3 weeks
** 5 FU 500 mg/m^2 + Doxorubicin 50 mg/m^2 + cyclophosphamide 500 mg/ m^2, day 1 every 3 weeks
*** 20 mg/day for 5 years

Update:

1042 patients recruited as of March 2003.

Title: A multicenter phase III randomized trial to compare the sequential and the concomitant administration of doxurubicin and docetaxel, as first line chemotherapy treatment for metastatic breast disease. GEICAM 9903

Coordinator: E. Alba
Servicio de Oncología Médica
Hospital U. Virgen de la Victoria
Colonia Santa Inés s/n
29010 MÁLAGA
SPAIN
Email: oncologia98@yahoo.com

Summary:
- Opened in December 1999
- Accrual completed with 144 patients
- Presented (Proceedings) at the 38th ASCO Annual Meeting

Objective:

To compare the hematological toxicity and efficacy of sequential vs concomitant administration of doxorubicin and docetaxel as metastatic breast cancer first-line treatment.

Scheme: *Randomization:*

- **Arm A:** sequential treatment with doxorubicin (A) (75 mg/m^2/q21d) and docetaxel (T) (100 mg/m^2/q21d). Patients with previous anthracyclines received A $\times$ 2 followed by T $\times$ 4. Patients without previous anthracyclines received A $\times$ 3 followed by T $\times$ 3.
- **Arm B:** concomitant treatment with A (50 mg/m^2) plus T (75 mg/m^2) q21d for 3 cycles, followed by 3 cycles of T (100 mg/m^2/q21d) in patients with previous anthracyclines, or by A plus T (50 mg/m^2 plus 75 mg/m^2) q21d for 3 cycles in patients without previous anthracyclines.

Update:

Publication of results is expected in 2003.

GEICAM

Title: A multicenter phase III randomized trial comparing 5-fluorouracil with epirubicin and cyclophosphamide (FEC) vs 5-fluorouracil with epirubicin and cyclophosphamide (FEC) followed by weekly paclitaxel as adjuvant treatment of operable breast cancer patients with positive axillary lymph nodes.
GEICAM 9906

Coordinators: Rodríguez Lescure
Servicio de Oncología Médica
Hospital General U. De Elche
03203 ELCHE-ALICANTE
SPAIN

J.M. López Vega
Servicio de Oncología Médica
Hospital U. Marqués de Valdecilla
Av. De Valdecilla s/n
39008 SANTANDER
SPAIN
Email: onclvj@humv.es

E. Aranda
Servicio de Oncología Médica
H.U. Reina Sofía
Av. Menéndez Pidal, s/n
14004 CÓRDOBA
SPAIN

Summary:
- Opened in December 1999
- Accrual completed in May 2002: 1250 patients

Objective:

To determine the relative efficacy and toxicity of 5-fluorouracil with epirubicin and cyclophosphamide (FEC) vs 5-fluorouracil with epirubicin and cyclophosphamide (FEC) followed by weekly paclitaxel as chemotherapy for operable breast cancer patients with positive axillary lymph nodes.

Scheme:

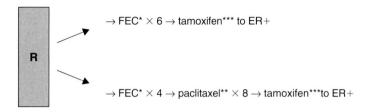

$\rightarrow$ FEC* $\times$ 6 $\rightarrow$ tamoxifen*** to ER+

$\rightarrow$ FEC* $\times$ 4 $\rightarrow$ paclitaxel** $\times$ 8 $\rightarrow$ tamoxifen***to ER+

* 5-Fluorouracil 600 mg/m2 + Epirubicin 90 mg/m2 + cyclophosphamide 600 mg/m2, day 1 every 3 weeks (6 cycles).
** 5FU 600 mg/m2 + Epirubicin 90 mg/m2 + cyclophosphamide 600 mg/m2, day 1 every 3 weeks (4 cycles) followed by paclitaxel 100 mg/m2 day 1 every week (8 weeks).
*** 20 mg/day for 5 years

Update:

First interim efficacy analysis planned in December 2003.

GEICAM

Title: An open, multicenter randomized phase IV trial for the administration of pamidronate to breast cancer patients with bone metastatic disease. GEICAM 2000-01

Coordinators: A. Lluch
Servicio de Oncología Médica
Hospital Clínico U. De Valencia
Av. Blasco Ibáñez, 17
46010 VALENCIA
SPAIN
Email: ana.lluch@uv.es

A. Barnadas i Molins
Servicio de Oncología Médica
Hospital Germans Trias i Pujol
Cta. Canyet s/n
8915 BADALONA-BARCELONA
SPAIN
Email: barnadas@ns.hugtip.scs.es

Summary:
- Opened in May 2000
- Accrual completed in December 2002 with 150 patients

Objective:

To compare continous administration of pamidronate for 18 months vs administration of aredia for 6 months followed by six months without treatment followed by administration of pamidronate for 6 months, to evaluate differences in time to first skeletal bone event in both arms.

Scheme: *Randomization:*

Arm A: Pamidronate 90 mg every 3–4 weeks for 18 months.
Arm B: Pamidronate 90 mg every 3–4 weeks for 6 months, then, 6 months at rest, followed by pamidronate 90 mg every 3–4 weeks for 6 months.

Title: An open, multicenter phase II trial for the administration of bi-weekly vinorelbine and UFT to metastatic breast cancer patients. GEICAM 2000-02

Coordinator: A. Antón
Servicio de Oncología Médica
Hospital U. Miguel Servet
Av. Isabel La Católica 1,3
50009 ZARAGOZA
SPAIN
Email: aanton08@airtel.net

Summary:
- Opened in September 2000
- Target: 35 patients

Objective:

To evaluate the activity of the study drugs, in terms of response rate to treatment.

Scheme: Vinorelbine 30 mg/m2 day 1 every 2 weeks.
UFT 250 mg/m2/day every day for 2 weeks.
This is called a treatment course. The treatment will continue until disease progression or unacceptable toxicity.

Update:

Accrual 34 patients as of March 2003.

GEICAM

Title:　A randomized phase III treatment to compare the administration of vinorelbine vs vinorelbine plus gemcitabine in patients with metastatic breast cancer previously treated with anthracyclines and taxanes. GEICAM 2000-04

Coordinator:　M. Martin
Servicio de Oncología Médica
Hospital Clínico U. San Carlos
Prof Martín Lagos s/n
28040 MADRID
SPAIN
Email: mmartín@geicam.org

Summary:
- Opened in December 2000
- Target: 254 patients

Objective:

To compare progression free survival among treatment arms A and B in patients with metastatic breast cancer who have previously been treated with anthracyclines and taxanes.

Scheme:　*Randomization:*

Arm A: Vinorelbine 30 mg/m2 days 1 and 8, every 3 weeks.
Arm B: Vinorelbine 30 mg/m2 days 1 and 8, every 3 weeks.
Gemcitabine 1200 mg/m2 days 1 and 8, every 3 weeks.

Patients will receive study treatment until progression of the disease or unacceptable toxicity.

Update:

Accrual 105 patients as of March 2003.

Title: Maintenance phase III / IV study for the administration of Caelyx® vs no treatment, after induction chemotherapy for metastatic breast cancer disease.
GEICAM 2001-01

Coordinator: E. Alba
Servicio de Oncología Médica
Hospital U. Virgen de la Victoria
Colonia Santa Inés s/n
29010 MÁLAGA
SPAIN
Email: oncologia98@yahoo.com

Summary: • Opened in June 2002
• Target: 154 patients

Objective:

To evaluate time to disease progression after maintenance treatment with pegilated lyposomal doxorubicin (Caelyx®) in patients with complete or partial response, or stable disease, vs non-maintenance treatment.

Scheme:

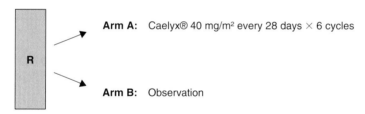

Arm A: Caelyx® 40 mg/m² every 28 days × 6 cycles

Arm B: Observation

Update:

Number of registered patients 59 as of March 2003.
Accrual 9 patients as of March 2003.

GEICAM

Title: A multicenter, cross-over, randomized trial with exemestane vs anastrozole as first line hormonal treatment of postmenopausal women with metastatic breast cancer disease and positive hormone receptors. GEICAM 2001-03

Coordinator: A. Llombart
Servicio de Oncología Médica
Instituto Valenciano de Oncología
C / Prof Beltrán Vaguean 8,9,19
46009 VALENCIA
SPAIN
Email: allombart1@yahoo.com

Summary:
- Opened in June 2001
- Target: 100 patients

Objective:

To evaluate objective response rate.

Scheme:

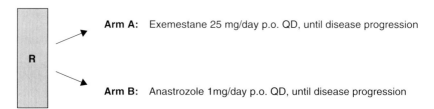

Arm A: Exemestane 25 mg/day p.o. QD, until disease progression

Arm B: Anastrozole 1mg/day p.o. QD, until disease progression

After disease progression, the investigator will decide the treatment cross-over whenever deemed appropriate.

Update:

Accrual 39 patients as of March 2003.

Title: Phase II study for weekly administration of trastuzumab with paclitaxel and cisplatin as first line chemotherapy treatment of metastatic breast cancer disease.
GEICAM 2001-04

Coordinator: E. Alba
Servicio de Oncología Médica
Hospital U. Virgen de la Victoria
Colonia Santa Inés s/n
29010 MÁLAGA
SPAIN
Email: oncologia98@yahoo.com

Summary:
- Opened in June 2001
- Target: 32 patients

Objective:

To evaluate objective response rate and toxicity of the chemotherapy scheme.

Scheme: 1 course of treatment = 3 weeks of treatment with paclitaxel and cisplatin + 4 weeks of treatment with trastuzumab. Courses will be repeated every 4 weeks.
- First (day 1): trastuzumab 4 mg/kg as loading dose and afterwards a maintenance weekly dose of 2 mg/kg.
- Second (day 2): paclitaxel 60 mg/m2 once a week $\times$ 3 weeks.
- Third (day 2): cisplatin 25 mg/m2 once a week $\times$ 3 weeks.

Study treatment will continue until disease progression.

Update:

Accrual 10 patients as of March 2003.

GEICAM

Title: A multicenter, open-lable, randomized phase III trial for the administration of zoledronate to patients with advanced breast cancer disease and non-symptomatic bone metastasis.
GEICAM 2001-05

Coordinator: A. Lluch
Servicio de Oncología Médica
Hospital Clínico U. De Valencia
Av. Blasco Ibáñez, 17
46010 VALENCIA
SPAIN
Email: ana.lluch@uv.es

A. Barnadas i Molins
Servicio de Oncología Médica
Hospital Germans Trias i Pujol
Cta. Canyet s/n
8915 BADALONA-BARCELONA
SPAIN
Email: barnadas@ns.hugtip.scs.es

Summary:
- Opened in April 2002
- Target: 224 patients

Objective:

To assess zoledronate efficacy (combined with hormone therapy or chemotherapy) to delay bone metastasis symptoms in breast cancer patients with at least one single bone disease location.

Scheme: *Randomization:*

Arm A: Zoledronate 4 mg every 3–4 weeks. Study treatment will be maintained until symptoms related to bone disease appear, or during 1 year (whichever occurs first).
Arm B: Patients will not receive any treatment with bisphosphonates until symptoms related to bone disease appear, or during 1 year (whichever occurs first).

Update:

Accrual 13 patients as of March 2003.

Title: A multicenter phase II trial to evaluate the administration of gemcitabine with doxorubicin and paclitaxel (GAT) as neo-adjuvant treatment of stage III disease breast cancer patients.
GEICAM 2002-01

Coordinators: P. Sánchez-Rovira
Servicio de Oncología Médica
Complejo Hospitalario Ciudad de Jaén
Av. Ejército Español s/n
23007 JAÉN
SPAIN
Email: oncomedhcj@amsystem.es

A. Antón
Servicio de Oncología Médica
Hospital U. Miguel Servet
Av. Isabel La Católica 1 y 3
50009 ZARAGOZA
SPAIN
Email: aanton08@airtel.net

Summary:
- Opened in January 2003
- Target: 43 patients

Objective:

To determine the rate of pathological complete response obtained with GAT combination of drugs in the neo-adjuvant treatment of stage III disease breast cancer patients.

Scheme:
A: doxorubicin 40 mg/m2, day 1 every other week
T: paclitaxel 150 mg/m2 day 2 every other week
G: gemcitabine 2000 mg/m2 day 2 every other week

This is defined a cycle. Each cycle is administered every 2 weeks, for a total of 6 cycles, prior to primary surgery of the breast.

GEICAM

Title: A phase II trial to evaluate the administration of doxorubicin with cyclophosphamide (AC) followed by weekly docetaxel (T) as neo-adjuvant treatment of stage II disease breast cancer patients.
GEICAM 2002-03

Coordinators: L. García Estévez
Servicio de Oncología Médica
Fundación Jiménez Díaz
Av. Reyes Católicos, 2
28040 MADRID
SPAIN
Email: lestevez@fjd.es

J.M. López Vega
Servicio de Oncología Médica
Hospital U. Marqués de Valdecilla
Av. Marqués de Valdecilla s/n
39008 SANTANDER
SPAIN
Email: onclvj@humv.es

Summary:
- Opened in January 2003
- Target: 61 patiens

Objective:

To determine the rate of pathological complete response (pCR) after induction treatment with doxorubicin and cyclophosphamide (AC) followed by weekly docetaxel in patients with operable breast cancer (stage II disease).

Scheme: **AC:** doxorubicin 60 mg/m^2 plus cyclophosphamide 600 mg/m^2 day 1 every 3 weeks (4 cycles), followed by
T: Docetaxel 36 mg/m^2 day 1, weekly, for 6 weeks.

A docetaxel cycle is defined as 6 weekly docetaxel infusions followed by 2 weeks without treatment (8 weeks). It is planned to administer 2 docetaxel cycles prior to primary breast surgery.

GOIRC

STUDIES

GOIRC

Title: Primary chemotherapy vs primary chemotherapy and endocrine therapy in operable breast carcinoma.
GOIRC – SANG 1B

Coordinator: Beatrice Di Blasio
Unità Operativa di Oncologia Medica
Azienda Ospedaliera di Parma
via Gramsci 14
43100 PARMA
ITALY
Tel: +39 0521 702682
Fax: +39 0521 995448
Email: bdiblasio@ao.pr.it

Summary:
- Opened in February 1998
- Target accrual: 270 patients

Objectives:

- To compare objective response rate and complete response rate to primary systemic treatment administering chemotherapy, or chemotherapy combined with endocrine therapy, in operable palpable breast cancer;
- To compare disease-free survival of treatment arms;
- To compare overall survival of treatment arms;
- To evaluate relationship between complete response and a few molecular markers prospectively determined with FNAB and immunocytochemistry.

Scheme:

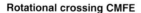

Rotational crossing CMFE
cyclophosphamide: 600 mg/m^2 d 1, 8;
methotrexate: 40 mg/m^2 d 1, 8;
fluorouracil: 600 mg/m^2 d 1, 8;
Epirubicin: 45 mg/m^2 d 1, 8;
every 28 days for 4 cycles
F, M, C, E are not administered on cycle 1, 2, 3, 4, respectively

Rotational crossing CMFE plus goserelin (in premenopause), **plus letrozole** 2.5 mg/day (in postmenopause)

Note: The endocrine therapy part of the study is administered until the end of adjuvant chemotherapy.

↓

Surgery

↓

Adjuvant chemotherapy: CMF for 3 cycles

↓

Tamoxifen: 20 mg/day for 5 years
(in ER+ and/or Pg R+ patients to be started at the end of adjuvant chemotherapy and of endocrine theraphy, if any)

Note: Other chemotherapy combinations are accepted by a prospective decision of each individual participating unit, before randomization.

Update:

Study closed in November 2002 with an accrual of 125 patients.

GOIRC

Title: Conventional chemotherapy compared to experimental chemotherapy (rotational crossing CMFEV) as adjuvant treatment in patients with moderate-high-risk stage I or with stage II (1 to 9 positive nodes) breast carcinoma.
GOIRC – SANG 2B

Substudies: A. CMF for 6 cycles compared to rotational crossing CMFEV for 6 cycles as adjuvant treatment in patients with moderate-high-risk stage I or stage II (1 to 3 positive nodes);

B. Adriamycin for 4 cycles followed by CMF for 4 cycles compared to rotational crossing CMFEV for 6 cycles as adjuvant treatment in patients with stage II (4 to 9 positive nodes) breast carcinoma.

Coordinator: Beatrice Di Blasio
Unità Operativa di Oncologia Medica
Azienda Ospedaliera di Parma
via Gramsci 14
43100 PARMA
ITALY
Tel: +39 0521 702682
Fax: +39 0521 995448
Email: bdiblasio@ao.pr.it

Chairs: G. Cocconi
Medical Oncology Division
University Hospital
43100 PARMA
ITALY
Tel: +390 52199 1316 / 259571
Fax: +390 52199 5448
Email: oncologia@ao.pr.it

C. Boni
Medical Oncology Service
Azienda Ospedaliera
42100 REGGIO EMILIA
ITALY
Tel: +390 522 29 6546
Fax: +390 522 29 6604
Email: oncologia@asmn.re.it

M. Tonato
Medical Oncology Division
University Hospital
06122 PERUGIA
ITALY
Tel: +390 755 738 3456
Fax: +390 755 720 990
Email: oncmedpg@krenet.it

Summary:
- Opened in September 1994
- Target accrual: 480 patients, with reference to substudy A; no target for substudy B

Main objectives:

- To compare disease-free survival administering an adjuvant chemotherapy, presently considered as conventional (CMF or sequence A → CMF), with the experimental chemotherapy rotational crossing CMFEV;
- To compare overall survival of treatment arms.

Objectives of two prospectively planned subgroup analyses:

A.
- To compare disease-free survival administering CMF, or the rotational crossing CMFEV, in patients with high-risk stage I or with stage II (1 to 3 positive nodes);
- To compare overall survival of treatment arms;
- To compare toxicity of treatment arms.

B.
- To compare disease-free survival administering the sequence A for 4 cycles followed by CMF for 4 cycles, or the rotational crossing CMFEV for 6 cycles, in patients with stage II (4 to 9 positive nodes);
- To compare overall survival of treatment arms;
- To compare toxicity of treatment arms.

Scheme:

Substudy A

T_{1c}; N−, but with at least one unfavourable prognostic factor among hormone receptors, proliferative activity, histologic grade.
T_2-T_3; N−;
T_1-T_2-T_3; N+ (1 to 3 positive nodes)

CMF:
C: 600 mg/m^2 d 1, 8;
M: 40 mg/m^2 d 1, 8;
F: 600 mg/m^2 d 1, 8;
every 28 days for 6 cycles

R

Rotational crossing CMFEV
C: 600 mg/m^2 d 1, 8;
M: 40 mg/m^2 d 1, 8;
F: 600 mg/m^2 d 1, 8;
E (Epirubicin): 40 mg/m^2 d 1, 8
V (vincristine): 1.4 mg/m^2 d 1;
every 28 days for 6 cycles
(F, M, C are not administered on 1st and 4th, 2nd and 5th, 3rd and 6th cycle, respectively)

Substudy B
T_1-T_2-T_3; N+ (4 to 9 positives nodes)

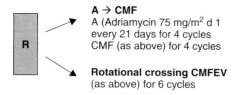

A → CMF
A (Adriamycin 75 mg/m² d 1
every 21 days for 4 cycles
CMF (as above) for 4 cycles

Rotational crossing CMFEV
(as above) for 6 cycles

For either substudy:

Tamoxifen, 20 mg per day, for 5 years, in all premenopausal ER+ patients and in all postmenopausal ER+ or ER– patients. Tamoxifen treatment is initiated at the end of chemotherapy.

Update:

Study closed on April 2000 with an accrual of 489 patients for substudy A and 142 patients for substudy B.

Title: Adjuvant chemotherapy with Adriamycin for 4 cycles followed by CMF for 4 cycles, or with three MVAC-like cisplatin (P)-containing combinations for 6 cycles in patients with very high-risk stage II breast carcinoma (10 or more positive nodes).
GOIRC – SANG 3B

Coordinator: Beatrice Di Blasio
Unità Operativa di Oncologia Medica
Azienda Ospedaliera di Parma
via Gramsci 14
43100 PARMA
ITALY
Tel: +39 0521 702682
Fax: +39 0521 995448
Email: bdiblasio@ao.pr.it

Summary:
- Opened in December 1993
- Target accrual: 100 patients

Objective:

To evaluate disease-free survival and overall survival in patients with very high-risk breast carcinoma treated with full dose Adriamycin (4 cycles) followed by CMF (4 cycles) or with MVAC-like (M on day 1, P on day 2) cisplatin and anthracycline containing combinations (6 cycles).

Scheme:

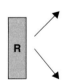

A → CMF
Adriamycin : 75 mg/m^2 day 1
every 21 days for 4 cycles
CMF: cyclophosphamide: 600 mg/m^2 days 1, 8; methotrexate: 40 mg/m^2 days 1, 8; fluorouracil: 600 mg/m^2 d 1, 8
every 28 days for 4 cycles

MPEpiE → MPEpiV → MPEMi
MPEpiE: methotrexate: 100 mg/m^2 days 1, 8 followed by L-leucovorin 7.5 mg every 6 hours, times 4, starting 24 h after M;
P (cisplatinum): 80 mg/m^2 d 2;
Epi (Epirubicin): 60 mg/m^2 day 1;
E (etoposide): 100 mg/m^2 d days 1, 2
every 21 days for 2 cycles
MPEpiV: M: as above;
P: as above;
Epi: as above;
V (vincristine): 1,4 mg/m^2 days 1, 8
every 21 days for 2 cycles
MPEMi: M: as above;
P: as above;
E: 120 mg/m^2 days 1, 2;
Mi (Mitomycin): 6 mg/m^2 day 1;
every 21 days for 2 cycles

Tamoxifen, 20 mg daily, for 5 years in premenopausal ER+ and in ER+ and ER postmenopausal patients, beginning at the end of chemotherapy.

Update:

The study was closed in April 2001 with an accrual of 90 patients.

GONO MIG

STUDIES

GONO MIG

Title: Standard CEF vs accelerated CEF as adjuvant chemotherapy in node-positive or high-risk node-negative (T > 2 cm, age < 35 yrs, G3, negative hormone receptors or high TL1 or S-phase) breast cancer. A phase III randomized trial.
MIG-1

Coordinator: Marco Venturini
Istituto Nazionale per la Ricerca sul Cancro
Largo R. Benzi 10
16132 GENOVA
ITALY
Tel: +39 010 5600 666
Fax: +39 010 5600 850
Email: marco.venturini@istge.it

Summary:
- Closed in June 1997 (opened in November 1992)
- Target accrual: 1200 patients

Objective:

To evaluate overall survival and disease-free survival in early breast cancer patients treated with standard CEF or accelerated CEF as adjuvant chemotherapy.

Scheme:

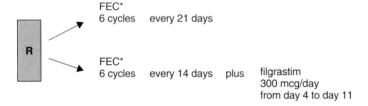

FEC*
6 cycles   every 21 days

FEC*
6 cycles   every 14 days   plus   filgrastim
300 mcg/day
from day 4 to day 11

* CYCLO 600 mg/m^2 + Epi ADM 60 mg/m^2 + 5FU 600 mg/m^2

Update:

Closed in June 1997.
Patients randomized: 1214.

Title: Epirubicin plus paclitaxel vs cyclophosphamide, Epirubicin and
             5-fluorouracil as adjuvant chemotherapy in node-positive breast cancer
             patients. A phase III randomized study.
             MIG-5

Coordinator: Marco Venturini
             Divisione di Oncologia Medica I
             Istituto Nazionale per la Ricera sul Cancro
             Largo Rosanna Benzi 10
             16132 GENOVA
             ITALY
             Tel: +390 10 5600 666
             Fax: +390 10 5600 850
             Email: marco.venturini@istge.it

Summary: • Opened in November 1996
             • Target accrual: 1000 patients

             Objective:

             To evaluate overall survival and disease-free survival in early breast cancer
             patients treated with Epirubicin plus paclitaxel or CEF as adjuvant
             chemotherapy.

Scheme:

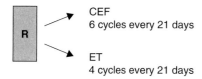

CEF
6 cycles every 21 days

ET
4 cycles every 21 days

CEF = cyclo 600 mg/m^2 + Epi ADM 60 mg/m^2 + 5FU 600 mg/m^2
ET = ADM 90 mg/m^2 + paclitaxel 175 mg/m^2 (3-hour infusion)

Update:

Closed January 2001.
1055 patients recruited.

IBCSG

STUDIES

IBCSG

Title: Adjuvant therapy in pre- and perimenopausal patients with node-negative breast cancer. Observation vs LH–RH analogue or CMF vs CMF + LN–RH analogue.
IBCSG trial VIII

Chair: M. Castiglione
IBCSG Coordinating Center
Effingerstr. 40
CH-3008 BERN
SWITZERLAND
Tel: +41 31 389 9391
Fax: +41 31 389 9392
Email: monica.castiglione@ibcsg.org

Summary:
- Closed in October 1999 (opened in May 1990)
- Target accrual: 1200 patients

Objectives:

- To determine whether the use of an LH-RH analogue following 6 months of CMF chemotherapy reduces relapse and prolongs survival as compared to the use of either a 2-year administration of an LH-RH analogue alone or the use of 6 months of CMF alone;
- To investigate the patients' perceptions on well-being and coping during adjuvant treatment, after therapy but before relapse, and after relapse.

Scheme:

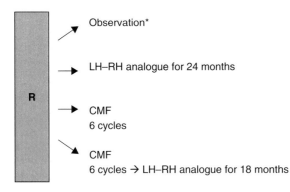

Observation*

LH–RH analogue for 24 months

CMF
6 cycles

CMF
6 cycles → LH–RH analogue for 18 months

*Observation arm dropped in April 1992

Update:

Trial closed October 1999.
Total patients randomized: 1111.

Title: Adjuvant therapy in node-negative postmenopausal patients with node-negative breast cancer. Tamoxifen vs CMF + Tamoxifen.
IBCSG trial IX

Chair: M. Castiglione
IBCSG Coordinating Center
Effingerstr. 40
CH-3008 BERN
SWITZERLAND
Tel: +41 31 389 9391
Fax: +41 31 389 9392
Email: monica.castiglione@ibcsg.org

Summary: • Closed in August 1999 (opened in October 1988)
• Target accrual: 1600 patients

Objectives:

• To evaluate if the addition of three cycles of initial chemotherapy to adjuvant tamoxifen improves outcome;
• To evaluate quality of life.

Scheme:

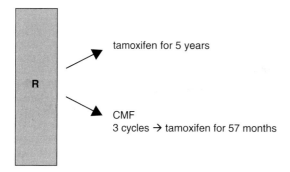

R

tamoxifen for 5 years

CMF
3 cycles → tamoxifen for 57 months

Update:

Trial closed 1 August 1999.
1715 patients randomized.

IBCSG

Title: Surgical therapy with or without axillary node clearance for breast cancer in
elderly patients who receive adjuvant therapy with tamoxifen.
IBCSG trial 10-93

Chair: D. Crivellari
Centro di Riferimento Oncologico Aviano
Inst. di Ricovero e Cura a Carattere Scientifico
Via Pedemonta Occ. 12
33081 AVIANO
ITALY
Tel: +390 434 659 316 / 659 206
Fax: +390 434 652 182
Email: dcrivellari@cro.it

C.M. Rudenstam
Bohusgatan 26
S-41139 GOTHENBURG
SWEDEN
Tel: +46 31 164 511
Fax: +46 31 602 172
Email: c-m.rudenstam@telia.com

Summary: • Opened in May 1993
• Closed December 2002
• Target accrual: 1020 patients

Objectives:

• To assess the relevance of an axillary node dissection in elderly patients, all
of whom receive adjuvant systemic therapy with tamoxifen, in terms of
disease-free survival, ipsilateral axillary events, occurrence of
postmastectomy (post primary surgery) syndrome, systemic disease-free
survival, overall survival, and toxic effects;
• To assess quality of life.

Scheme:

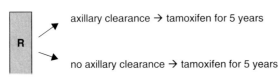

axillary clearance → tamoxifen for 5 years

R

no axillary clearance → tamoxifen for 5 years

Update:

473 patients randomized by IBCSG.

Title: Adjuvant therapy for premenopausal patients with node-positive breast cancer who are suitable for endocrine therapy alone.
IBCSG trial 11-93

Chairs: B. Thürlimann
Medizinische Klinik C
Kantonsspital
CH-9007 ST GALLEN
SWITZERLAND
Tel: +41 71 494 1111
Fax: +41 71 494 2878
Email: beat.thuerlimann@kssg.ch

M. Castiglione
IBCSG Coordinating Center
Effingerstr. 40
CH-3008 BERN
SWITZERLAND
Tel: +41 31 389 9391
Fax: +41 31 389 9392
Email: monica.castiglione@ibcsg.org

Summary:
- Closed November 1998 (opened in May 1993)
- Target accrual: 400 patients

Objectives:

- To evaluate if the addition of chemotherapy (AC × 4) to endocrine therapy alone (oophorectomy, tamoxifen) improves outcome;
- To assess quality of life.

Scheme:

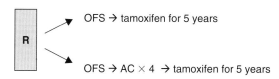

R

OFS → tamoxifen for 5 years

OFS → AC × 4 → tamoxifen for 5 years

Update:

Study closed November 1998.
Total number of patients randomized: 174.

IBCSG

Title: Adjuvant therapy for post/perimenopausal patients with node-positive breast cancer who are suitable for endocrine therapy alone.
IBCSG trial 12-93

Chairs: E. Simoncini
Oncologica Medica
Spedali Civili
Piazzale Spedali Civili 1
25100 BRESCIA
ITALY
Tel: +39 03 0399 5410
Fax: +39 03 0370 0017

A. Goldhirsch
Oncology Institute of Southern Switzerland
Ospedale Regionale di Lugano (Civico)
Via Tesserete 46
CH-6900 LUGANO
SWITZERLAND
Tel: +41 91 811 6515
Fax: +41 91 811 6517
Email: agoldhirsch@sakk.ch

Summary:
- Closed in August 1999 (opened in May 1993)
- Target accrual: 960 patients

Objectives:

- To evaluate if toremifene is equally effective as tamoxifen in controlling breast cancer;
- To assess quality of life.

Scheme:

Stratify:
- primary therapy (sx, XRT plan)
- institution
- Adjuvant CT planned?

Yes

No

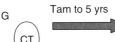

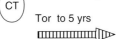

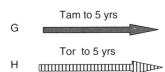

Tam to 5 yrs

Tor to 5 yrs

Tam to 5 yrs

Tor to 5 yrs

Update:

Trial closed August 1999.
452 patients randomized.

Title: Adjuvant therapy for premenopausal patients with node-positive breast cancer who are not suitable for endocrine therapy alone.
IBCSG trial 13-93

Chairs: A. Coates
Royal Prince Alfred Hospital
E 9 Special Unit
Camperdown SYDNEY
AUSTRALIA
Tel: +61 2 9515 6123
Fax: +61 2 9515 1546
Email: alancoates@cancer.org.au

M. Castiglione
IBCSG Coordinating Center
Effingerstr. 40
CH-3008 BERN
SWITZERLAND
Tel: +41 31 389 9391
Fax: +41 31 389 9392
Email: monica.castiglione@ibcsg.org

Summary:
- Closed August 1999 (opened in May 1993)
- Target accrual: 1225 patients

Objectives:

- To evaluate if a 16 week treatment-free interval between two sequential chemotherapy regimens (AC × 4, CMF × 3) improves outcome;
- To evaluate if tamoxifen maintenance following chemotherapy improves outcome;
- To assess quality of life.

Scheme:

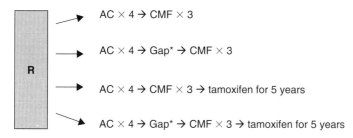

R

AC × 4 → CMF × 3

AC × 4 → Gap* → CMF × 3

AC × 4 → CMF × 3 → tamoxifen for 5 years

AC × 4 → Gap* → CMF × 3 → tamoxifen for 5 years

* Gap = 16 week treatment-free interval

Update:

Trial closed August 1999.
1294 patients randomized.

IBCSG

Title: Adjuvant therapy for post- perimenopausal patients with node-positive breast cancer who are not suitable for endocrine therapy alone. IBCSG trial 14-93

Chairs: O. Pagani
Instituto Oncologico Suizz. Italiano (IOSI)
Ospedale Beata Vergine
6850 MENDRISIO
SWITZERLAND
Tel: +41 91 811 3111
Fax: +41 92 811 3038
Email: opagani@siak.ch

A. Goldhirsch
Oncology Institute of Southern Switzerland
Ospedale Regionale di Lugano (Civico)
CH-6900 LUGANO
SWITZERLAND
Tel: +41 91 811 6515
Fax: +41 91 811 6517
Email: agoldhirsch@sakk.ch

Summary:
- Closed in August 1999 (opened in May 1993)
- Target accrual: 884 patients

Objectives:

- To evaluate if a 16 week treatment-free interval between two sequential chemotherapy regimens (AC × 4, CMF × 3) improves outcome;
- To evaluate if toremifene is equally effective as tamoxifen in controlling breast cancer following completion of all chemotherapy;
- To assess quality of life.

Scheme:

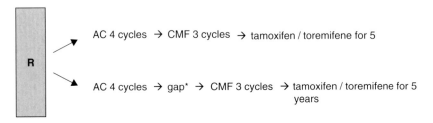

AC 4 cycles → CMF 3 cycles → tamoxifen / toremifene for 5

AC 4 cycles → gap* → CMF 3 cycles → tamoxifen / toremifene for 5 years

* gap = 16 week treatment-free interval

Update:

Trial closed August 1999.
969 patients randomized.

Title: High dose EC × 3 supported by PBSC vs EC / AC × 4 followed by CMF as adjuvant treatment for high risk operable stage II and stage III breast cancer in premenopausal and young postmenopausal (less than 65 years) patients. IBCSG trial 15-95

Chair: R. Basser
45 Poplar Road
PARKVILLE
VIC 3052
AUSTRALIA
Tel: +61 3 9389 1569
Fax: +61 3 9388 2351

Summary: • Opened in July 1995
• Target accrual: 300 patients

Objectives:

• To evaluate if a regimen of high-dose chemotherapy (EC × 3) improves outcome when compared with standard dose chemotherapy (AC × 4 → CMF × 3) for patients with a high-risk of recurrence;
• To evaluate quality of life.

Scheme:

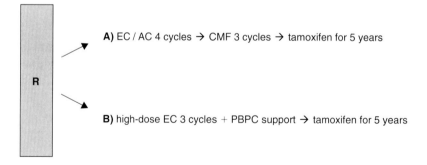

A) EC / AC 4 cycles → CMF 3 cycles → tamoxifen for 5 years

B) high-dose EC 3 cycles + PBPC support → tamoxifen for 5 years

Update:

Trial closed March, 2000
344 patients randomized.

IBCSG

Title: Adjuvant therapy for postmenopausal patients with operable breast cancer who have estrogen receptor or progesterone receptor positive tumors. Tamoxifen vs letrozole vs tamoxifen followed by letrozole vs letrozole followed by tamoxifen.
BIG 01-98 / IBCSG 18-98

Chair: B. Thuerlimann
Senologie Zentrum Ostschweiz
Kantonsspital
ST GALLEN
SWITZERLAND
Tel: +41 71 494 2065
Fax: +41 71 494 6368
Email: beat.thuerlimann@kssg.ch

Summary:
- Date of activation: March 1998
- Targeted accrual: over 7900 patients

Objective:

To compare disease-free survival, overall survival, and distant disease-free survival.

Scheme:

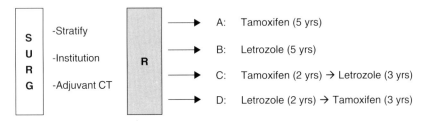

Update:

- Main study closed May 2003. Total accural: 8029.

Substudies:
- Bone Mineral Density substudy closed February 2003.
- General Safety / Lipid Profile substudy closed February 2003.

Title: Maintenance chemotherapy in hormone non-responsive breast cancer: Low-dose Cytotoxics as "Anti-angiogenesis Treatment" following Adjuvant Induction Chemotherapy for Patients with ER-negative and PgR-negative Breast Cancer.
IBCSG trial 22-00

Chair: Dr Marco Colleoni
European Institute of Oncology, EIO
Dept of Medicine: Division of Medical Oncology
Via Ripamonti 435
I-20141 MILANO
ITALY
Tel: +39 02 574 89 502
Fax:+39 02 57489 457
E-mail: marco.colleoni@ieo.it

Summary: • Date of activation: November 2000
• Target accrual: 900

Objective:

To evaluate the efficacy of a low-dose chemotherapy regimen, hypothesized to have antiangiogenic activity, administered following a standard chemotherapy program in patients whose tumors are not endocrine therapy-responsive.

Scheme:

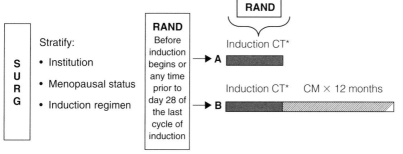

* Approved Induction CT Regimens.
  Please refer to the protocol for details.

IBCSG

Title: A randomized trial of axillary dissection vs no axillary dissection for patients with clinically node negative breast cancer and micrometastases in the sentinel node.
IBCSG trial 23-01

Chairs: Dr Viviana Galimberti
Instituto Europeo di Oncologia
Via Ripamonti 435
I-20141 MILANO
ITALY
Tel: +39 02 57489 717
Fax: +39 02 57489 780
Email: viviana.galimberti@ieo.it

Dr Stefano Zurrida
Instituto Europeo di Oncologia
Via Ripamonti 435
I-20141 MILANO
ITALY
Tel: +39 02 57489 608 / 215
Email: stefano.zurrida@ieo.it

Prof Umberto Veronesi
Instituto Europeo di Oncologia
Via Ripamonti 435
I-20141 MILANO
ITALY
Tel: +39 02 57224 / 215
Fax: +39 02 57489 210
Email: umberto.veronesi@ieo.it

Summary: • Date of activation: December 10th, 2001
• Target accrual: 1960 patients

Objective:

To compare axillary dissection vs no axillary dissection in terms of disease-free survival in patients with one micrometastasis in a sentinel node.

Scheme:

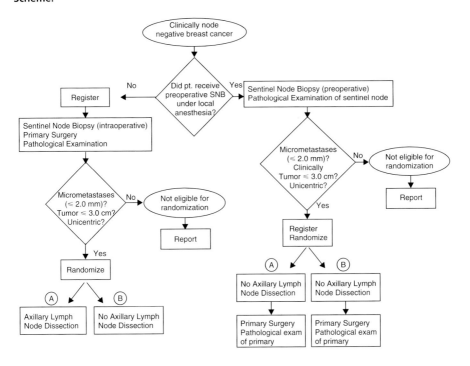

IBCSG

Title: Suppression of Ovarian Function Trial (SOFT)
BIG 2-02 / IBCSG trial 24-02

Chairs: **BIG:** Dr Prue Francis
Peter MacCallum Cancer Institute
St Andrews Place
3002 EAST MELBOURNE, VIC
AUSTRALIA
Tel: +61 3 965 61 700
Fax: +61 3 965 61 408
Email: pfrancis@petermac.unimelb.edu.au

US Intergroup: Dr Gini Fleming
University of Chicago Medical Center
Section of Hematology / Oncology
5841 South Maryland Ave, MC 2115
CHICAGO, IL 60637-1470
USA
Tel: +1 773 702 6712
Fax: +1 773 702 0963
Email: gfleming@medicine.bsd.uchicago.edu

Summary: • Planned activation date: August 2003
• Target accrual: 3000 patients

Objectives:

• To evaluate the role of ovarian function suppression and the role of exemestane as adjuvant therapies for premenopausal women with endocrine responsive breast cancer;
• To assess quality of life.

Scheme:

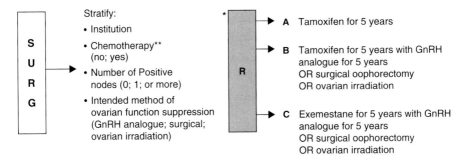

Stratify:
- Institution
- Chemotherapy** (no; yes)
- Number of Positive nodes (0; 1; or more)
- Intended method of ovarian function suppression (GnRH analogue; surgical; ovarian irradiation)

R

A Tamoxifen for 5 years

B Tamoxifen for 5 years with GnRH analogue for 5 years
OR surgical oophorectomy
OR ovarian irradiation

C Exemestane for 5 years with GnRH analogue for 5 years
OR surgical oophorectomy
OR ovarian irradiation

* Patients may have received tamoxifen or aromatase inhibitor prior to randomization
** Any standard chemotherapy

IBCSG

Title: Tamoxifen and Exemestane Trial (TEXT)
BIG 3-02 / IBCSG trial 25-02

Chair: **BIG:** Dr Olivia Pagani
Oncology Institute of Southern Switzerland
Ospedale Beata Vergine
6850 MENDRISIO
SWITZERLAND
Tel: +41 91 646 01 01
Fax: +41 91 646 02 52
Email: opagani@siak.ch

US Intergroup: Dr Barbara Walley
Tom Baker Cancer Centre
1331 – 29 St. N.W.
CALGARY, ALBERTA
CANADA
Tel: +1 403 670 1013
Fax: +1 403 283 1651
Email: bwalley@CancerBoard.ab.ca

Summary: • Planned activation date: August 2003
• Target accrual: 1845 patients

Objectives:

• To evaluate the role of exemestane plus GnRH analogue as adjuvant therapy for premenopausal women with endocrine responsive breast cancer;
• To assess quality of life.

Scheme:

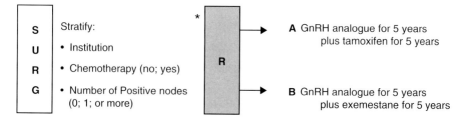

* Randomization prior to receiving any adjuvant systemic therapy

Title: Premenopausal Endocrine Responsive Chemotherapy Trial (PERCHE)
BIG 4-02 / IBCSG trial 26-02

Chair: **BIG:** (to be dermined)

BIG: US Intergroup: Dr Edith A. Perez, MD
Mayo Clinic Jacksonville
4500 San Pablo Road S
JACKSONVILLE, FL 32224-1865
USA
Tel: +1 904 953 2000
Fax: +1 904 953 2315
Email: perez.edith@mayo.edu

Summary:
- Planned activation date: August 2003
- Target accrual: 1750 patients

Objectives:

- To evaluate the role of chemotherapy as adjuvant therapy for premenopausal women with endocrine responsive breast cancer who receive endocrine therapy;
- To assess quality of life.

Scheme:

Stratify:

S U R G

- Institution
- Number of positive nodes (0; 1; or more)
- Intended initial method of ovarian function suppression (GnRH analogue × 5; surgical oophorectomy; ovarian irradiation
- Intended chemotherapy, if randomized to receive it (not containing anthracycline nor taxane; containing anthracycline or taxane)
- Intended endocrine agent (tamoxifen, exemestane; selected by randomization in the TEXT study)

*

R

A Chemotherapy
plus OFS
plus tamoxifen
or exemestane
for 5 years

B OFS
plus tamoxifen
or exemestane
for 5 years

* Randomization prior to receiving any adjuvant systemic therapy
OFS = Ovarian Function Suppression

IBCSG

Title: Chemotherapy for Radically Resected Loco-regional Relapse
BIG 1-02 / IBCSG trial 27-02

Chairs: PD Dr Stefan Aebi
Institute of Medical Oncology
Inselspital
3010 BERN
SWITZERLAND
Tel: +41 31 632 4114
Fax: +41 31 382 1237
Email: stefan.aebi@insel.ch

Dr Helmut F. Rauschecker
Westermayer 18
83022 ROSENHEIM
GERMANY
Tel: +49 80 3121 9990
Fax: +49 80 3138 1367
Email: rauschecker@t-online.de

Summary: • Date of activation: July 2002
• Target accrual: 977 patients

Objective:

To evaluate the efficacy of adjuvant chemotherapy after radical local
treatment of a first loco-regional recurrence of breast cancer.

Scheme:

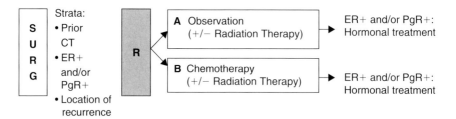

IBIS

STUDIES

IBIS

Title: An international multi-centre study of anastrozole vs placebo in postmenopausal women at increased risk of breast cancer. IBIS-II (Prevention). BIG 05-02a

Chairs: J. Cuzick
Cancer Research UK Department of Epidemiology, Mathematics and Statistics
Wolfson Institute of Preventive Medicine
Charterhouse Square
LONDON EC1M 6BQ
UNITED KINGDOM
Tel: +44 207 882 6196
Fax: +44 207 882 6252
Email: jack.cuzick@cancer.org.uk

J.F. Forbes
Dept of Surgical Oncology
University of Newcastle
Newcastle Mater Misericordiae Hospital
Locked bag 7
HUNTER REGION MAIL CENTRE, NSW 2310
AUSTRALIA
Tel: +61 2 4921 1155
Fax: +61 2 4929 1966
Email: john.forbes@anzbctg.newcastle.edu.au

A. Howell
CRC Medical Oncology
Christie Hospital
Wilmslow Road
Winthington
MANCHESTER M20 4BX
UNITED KINGDOM
Tel: +44 161 446 8037
Fax: +44 161 446 8000 / 3299
Email: maria.parker@christie-tr.nwest.nhs.uk

Summary:
- To open in 2003
- Target accrual: 6000

Objectives:

Primary:
To determine if anastrozole is effective in preventing breast cancer in postmenopausal women at increased risk of the disease.

Secondary:
- To examine the role of anastrozole in preventing oestrogen receptor positive breast cancer;
- To examine the effect of anastrozole on breast cancer mortality;
- To examine the effect of anastrozole on other cancers, cardiovascular disease, fracture rates, and non-breast cancer deaths;
- To examine tolerability and acceptability of side effects experience by women on the study.

Scheme:

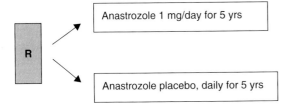

R → Anastrozole 1 mg/day for 5 yrs

R → Anastrozole placebo, daily for 5 yrs

Update:

Opened Spring 2003.

IBIS

Title: An international multi-centre study of tamoxifen vs anastrozole in postmenopausal women with Ductal Carcinoma in situ IBIS-II (DCIS). BIG 05-02b

Chairs: J. Cuzick
Cancer Research UK Department of Epidemiology, Mathematics and Statistics
Wolfson Institute of Preventive Medicine
Charterhouse Square
LONDON EC1M 6BQ
UNITED KINGDOM
Tel: +44 207 882 6196
Fax: +44 207 882 6252
Email: jack.cuzick@cancer.org.uk

J.F. Forbes
Dept of Surgical Oncology
University of Newcastle
Newcastle Mater Misericordiae Hospital
Locked bag 7
HUNTER REGION MAIL CENTRE, NSW 2310
AUSTRALIA
Tel: +61 2 4921 1155
Fax: +61 2 4929 1966
Email: john.forbes@anzbctg.newcastle.edu.au

A. Howell
CRC Medical Oncology
Christie Hospital
Wilmslow Road
Winthington
MANCHESTER M20 4BX
UNITED KINGDOM
Tel: +44 161 446 8037
Fax: +44 161 446 8000 / 3299
Email: maria.parker@christie-tr.nwest.nhs.uk

Summary:
- To open in 2003
- Target accrual: 4000

Objectives:

Primary:
To determine if anastrozole is at least as effective as tamoxifen in local control and prevention of contralateral disease in women with locally excised DCIS.

Secondary:
- To compare the effectiveness of tamoxifen and anastrozole according to the receptor status of the primary or recurrent cancer;
- To examine the rate of breast cancer recurrence and new contralateral tumours after cessation of tamoxifen or anastrozole;
- To examine the effect of tamoxifen vzs anastrozole on breast cancer mortality;
- To examine the effect of tamoxifen and anastrozole on other cancers, cardiovascular disease, fracture rates, and non-breast cancer deaths;
- To examine tolerability and acceptability of side effects experience by women on the study;

Scheme:

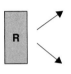

Tamoxifen 20 mg + Anastrozole placebo, daily for 5 yrs

Anastrozole 1 mg + Tamoxifen placebo, daily for 5 yrs

Update:

Opened Spring 2003.

ICCG

STUDIES

ICCG

Title: Epirubicin plus tamoxifen vs tamoxifen alone in postmenopausal node-positive primary breast cancer.
C/4/87

Coordinator: J. Wils
St Laurentius Ziekenhuis
NL-6043 CV ROERMOND
THE NETHERLANDS
Tel: +31 475 38 24 66
Fax: +31 475 38 24 36

Summary:
- Closed in April 1998 (opened in September 1989)
- Target accrual: 694 patients

Objectives:

- Disease-free survival;
- Survival.

Scheme:

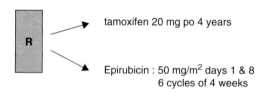

tamoxifen 20 mg po 4 years

Epirubicin : 50 mg/m^2 days 1 & 8
6 cycles of 4 weeks

tamoxifen 20 mg po 4 years

Update:

Study closed April 1998.
648 patients randomized.
Long term follow up ongoing.
Publication: Journal of Clinical Oncology, July 1999; 17(7): 1988–1998.

Title: Adjuvant cyclophosphamide, methotrexate and 5-fluorouracil (CMF) vs 5-fluorouracil, Epirubicin and cyclophosphamide (FEC) in women with node-negative, poor-risk primary breast cancer.
C/6/89

Coordinator: M. Marty
Hôpital St Louis
Service d'Oncologie
Med et Maladies du Sein
75475 PARIS Cedex 10
FRANCE
Tel: +33 1 42 499 938
Fax: +33 1 42 431 470

Summary:
- Opened in February 1990
- Target accrual: no target accrual but interim analysis after 600 patients

Objectives:

- Disease-free survival;
- Overall survival.

Scheme:

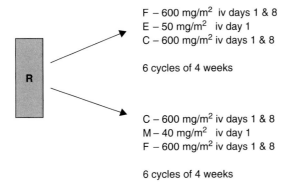

$F - 600$ mg/m^2 iv days 1 & 8
$E - 50$ mg/m^2 iv day 1
$C - 600$ mg/m^2 iv days 1 & 8

6 cycles of 4 weeks

$C - 600$ mg/m^2 iv days 1 & 8
$M - 40$ mg/m^2 iv day 1
$F - 600$ mg/m^2 iv days 1 & 8

6 cycles of 4 weeks

Update:

Study closed to recruitment on 1 August 2000.
Number of patients accrued: 950.
Active follow up continues.

ICCG

Title: Adjuvant FEC50 vs FEC75 with or without the additional benefit of sequential hormone therapy (HT) in node-positive premenopausal primary breast cancer.
C/9/91

Coordinator: M. Marty
Hôpital St Louis
Service d'Oncologie
Med et Maladies du Sein
75475 PARIS Cedex 10
FRANCE
Tel: +33 1 42 499 938
Fax: +33 1 42 431 470

Summary:
- Opened in March 1992
- Target accrual: 720 patients

Objectives:

- Disease-free survival;
- Overall survival.

Scheme:

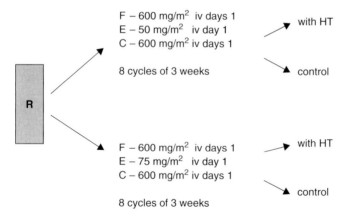

Update:

Study closed to recruitment on 1 August 2000.
Number of patients accrued: 785.
Active follow up continues.

Title: High-dose therapy with PBCS support in primary breast cancer.
C/10/92 – C/32/96

Coordinator: R.C. Coombes
Dept of Medical Oncology
Imperial College London
Charing Cross Campus
Fulham Palace Road
LONDON, W6 8RF
UNITED KINGDOM
Tel: +44 (0)208 383 5831
Fax: +44 (0)208 741 0731
Email: c.coombes@imperial.ac.uk

Summary:
- Opened in July 1993
- Target accrual: 230 patients

Objectives:

- Disease-free survival;
- Overall survival.

Scheme:

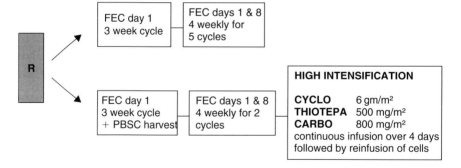

Update:

Study closed to recruitment on 28 September 2001.
Number of patients accrued: 281.
Active follow up continues.

ICCG

Title: Randomized double-blind trial in postmenopausal women with primary breast cancer who have received adjuvant tamoxifen for 2–3 years, comparing subsequent adjuvant exemestane treatment with further tamoxifen.
BIG 02-97 / Study no. 96 OEXE 031-C/13/96

Coordinator: R.C. Coombes
Dept of Medical Oncology
Imperial College London
Charing Cross Campus
Fulham Palace Road
LONDON, W6 8RF
UNITED KINGDOM
Tel: +44 (0)208 383 5831
Fax: +44 (0)208 741 0731
Email: c.coombes@imperial.ac.uk

Summary:
- Opened in February 1998
- Target accrual: 1103 patients/arm

Objectives:

- To evaluate disease-free survival and overall survival in ER+ / unknown breast cancer patients treated either with tamoxifen or with exemestane after having received adjuvant tamoxifen for 2–3 years;
- To evaluate the incidence of contralateral breast cancer and the general long term tolerability of the regimens;
- To evaluate the tolerability of each regimen in terms of endometrial status, bone metabolism, lipid profile, coagulation profile and quality of life.

Scheme:

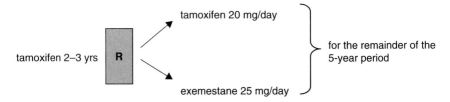

Quality of Life Sub Protocol –
A study to compare the quality of life of those patients allocated to tamoxifen with those allocated to exemestane, with the aim of determining efficacy, toxicity and overall general health and well being.

Endometrial Sub Protocol –
A study to assess endometrial ultrasound changes in postmenopausal patients receiving exemestane after 2-3 years of adjuvant tamoxifen compared to patients continuing on tamoxifen.

Bone Sub Protocol –
To compare bone mineral density (BMD) and metabolism in patients receiving exemestane with those receiving tamoxifen.

Update:

The main study closed to recruitment on 28 February 2003.
4743 patients recruited.

Quality of Life Study – Closed to recruitment on 31 December 2001.
581 patients recruited.

Endometrial Study – Closed to recruitment on 31 August 2001.
219 patients recruited.

Bone Study – Closed to recruitment on 28 February 2003.
206 patients recruited.

ICCG

Title: A multicentre randomized trial of sequential Epirubicin and docetaxel vs Epirubicin in node-positive postmenopausal breast cancer patients.
C/14/96

Coordinator: F. Erdkamp
Maaslandziekenhuis
Internal Medicine
Postbus 5500
NL-6130 MB SITTARD
THE NETHERLANDS
Tel: +31 46 459 7896
Fax: +31 46 459 7983

P.J. Hupperets
Dept of Internal Medicine
Division of Haematology-Oncology
University Hospital Maastricht
P.O. Box 5800
NL-6202 AZ MAASTRICHT
THE NETHERLANDS
Tel: +31 43 387 7025
Fax: +31 43 387 5006
Email: phu@sint.azm.nl

Summary:
- Opened in August 1997
- Target accrual: 800 patients

Objectives:

Primary:
- Disease-free survival;
- Overall survival.

Secondary:
- Incidence of thromboembolic events (selected centers).

Scheme:

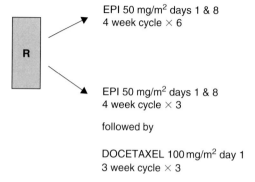

EPI 50 mg/m^2 days 1 & 8
4 week cycle $\times$ 6

EPI 50 mg/m^2 days 1 & 8
4 week cycle $\times$ 3

followed by

DOCETAXEL 100 mg/m^2 day 1
3 week cycle $\times$ 3

Update:

577 patients entered to date (July 2003).

ICCG

Study: A phase III multicentre double blind randomized trial of celecoxib vs placebo following chemotherapy in primary breast cancer patients. An intergroup study from the International Collaborative Cancer Group and the German Breast Group (GBG).
BIG 1-03 – ICCG / C/20/01 – GBG 27
(see also study description under GBG)

Coordinators: Prof R.C. Coombes
Director of ICCG Data Centre
ICCG Data Centre – Medical Oncology
Division of Medicine
Faculty of Medicine
Imperial College London
Charing Cross Campus
LONDON
Tel: +44 (0) 20 8846 1418
Fax: +44 (0) 20 8741 0731
Email: c.coombes@imperial.ac.uk

PD Dr med Gunter von Minckwitz
CEO, GBG Research GmbH
Co-Chair of the Celecoxib Study
Leiter der klinischen Prüfung
Klinikum der J.W. Goethe-Universitaet
Theodor-Stern-Kai 7
60590 FRANKFURT
GERMANY
Tel: +49 69 6301 7024
Fax: +49 69 6301 7938
Email: minckwitz@germanbreastgroup.de

Summary:
- Study due to open in September 2003
- Target accrual: 2590 patients

Primary aim:
To assess the disease-free survival (DFS) benefit of two years adjuvant therapy with the COX-2 inhibitor celecoxib compared with placebo in primary breast cancer patients.

Secondary aims:
- Overall survival;
- The toxicity associated with long term use of celecoxib in primary breast cancer patients;
- Cardiovascular mortality;
- The incidence of second primaries.

Scheme:

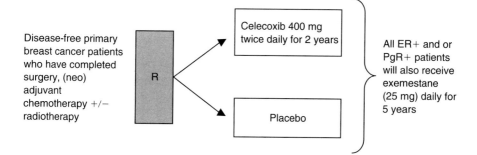

Disease-free primary breast cancer patients who have completed surgery, (neo) adjuvant chemotherapy +/− radiotherapy

R

Celecoxib 400 mg twice daily for 2 years

Placebo

All ER+ and or PgR+ patients will also receive exemestane (25 mg) daily for 5 years

Update:

Study will begin recruitment in September 2003.

ICR-CTSU

STUDIES

ICR-CTSU

Title: The NCRI Adjuvant Breast Cancer (ABC) Trial.
ISRCTN: 31514446

Clinical Coordinator: J. Yarnold
Royal Marsden Hospital NHS Trust
Downs Road
SUTTON
SURREY, SM2 5PT
UNITED KINGDOM
Tel: +44 20 8661 3891
Fax: +44 20 8661 3107
Email: john.yarnold@icr.ac.uk

Trial Coordinator: David Lawrence
Clinical Trials & Statistics Unit (ICR-CTSU)
Section of Epidemiology
The Institute of Cancer Research
Brookes Lawley Building
15 Cotswold Road
SUTTON
SURREY, SM2 5NG
UNITED KINGDOM
Email: david.Lawrence@icr.ac.uk

Summary: Opened in January 1993; closed in September 2000.

Objective:

To test whether adjuvant chemotherapy (CT) and/or ovarian suppression (OS) add to the benefits of tamoxifen in pre/perimenopausal women.

Scheme:

Treatment plan for individual patients (not randomized)	Additional treatment options (randomized)	
	±OS	±CT
Tamoxifen	434	1747
Tamoxifen + CT	1710	–
Tamoxifen + OS	–	244
TOTAL	2144	1991

* Patients in the double randomization (±CT ±OS) count twice

Substudies: • Biological predictors of therapeutic response
                     • Quality of Life

Update:

Study closed; 3854 patients recruited (2144 pre/peri-menopausal patients randomized to ±OS*, 637 pre/peri-menopausal patients randomized to ±CT* and 1354 postmenopausal patients randomized to ±CT. Total of 1991 patients randomized to ±CT).

ICR-CTSU

Title: The UK randomized trial of Hormone Replacement Therapy (HRT) in women with a history of early stage breast cancer.
ISRCTN: 29941643

Principal Clinical Investigators:
N. Sacks and J. Marsden
Royal Marsden Hospital
Fulham Road
LONDON
UNITED KINGDOM

Trial Coordinator:
C. Dawson
Clinical Trials & Statistics Unit (ICR-CTSU)
Section of Epidemiology,
The Institute of Cancer Research
Brookes Lawley Building
15 Cotswold Road
SUTTON
SURREY, SM2 5NG
UNITED KINGDOM
Tel: +44 208 722 4373
Fax: +44 208 770 7876
Email: claire.dawson@icr.ac.uk

Summary:
- Opened March 2002
- Target accrual: 3000

Objectives:

- To assess the effect of HRT on disease free survival and overall survival;
- The relief of menopausal symptoms and quality of life;
- Coronary heart disease, vascular events (i.e. thromboembolic, cerebrovascular) and osteoporotic fractures.

Scheme:
HRT arm*: If hysterectomised: unopposed oestrogen
If intact uterus: sequential combined therapy
continuous combined therapy

* choice and route of preparation will be determined by menopausal status and patient preference, where appropriate

No-HRT arm – advice on: practical measures
clonidine
evening primrose oil
health foods
complementary medicine (e.g., reflexology,
acupuncture, massage, meditation)

Low dose progesterones and phyto-oestrogen supplements are not
recommended

In both arms: preparation available for use for vaginal dryness

Update:

115 patients randomized to June 2003.

ICR-CTSU

Title: NCRI Standardisation of Breast Radiotherapy (START) Trial.
ISRCTN 59368779

Clinical Coordinator: J. Yarnold
Royal Marsden Hospital NHS Trust
Downs Road
SUTTON
SURREY, SM2 5PT
UNITED KINGDOM
Tel: +44 20 8661 3891
Fax: +44 20 8661 3107
Email: john.yarnold@icr.ac.uk

Trial Coordinator: Mark Sydenham
Clinical Trials and Statistics Unite (ICR-CTSU)
Section of Epidemiology
Institute of Cancer Research
Brookes Lawley Building
Cotswold Road
SUTTON
SURREY, SM2 5PT
UNITED KINGDOM
Tel: +44 20 8722 4104
Fax: +44 20 8770 7876
Email: mark.sydenham@icr.ac.uk

Summary:

- Opened January 1999; closed to recruitment October 2002.
- Target accrual: 2010 in Trial A (=670 per arm); 1840 in Trial B (=920 per arm).

Objective:

To test the effects of radiotherapy schedules using fraction sizes larger than 2.0 Gy in terms of locoregional tumour control, normal tissue responses, quality of life and economic consequences in women prescribed postoperative radiotherapy for early beast cancer.

Scheme:

Trial A

50 Gy / 25 Fractions (2.0 Gy) / 5 wks
vs 40 Gy / 15 Fractions (2.67 Gy) / 3 wks
vs 39 Gy / 13 Fractions (3.0 Gy) / 5 wks

Trial B

50 Gy / 25 Fractions (2.0 Gy) / 5 wks
vs 41.6 Gy / 13 Fractions (3.2 Gy) / wks

Substudies:

Accrual (end December 2002)	Trial A	Trial B	TOTAL
Quality of Life study	1127 *(600)*	1078 *(400)*	2205
Photographic assessments	1311 *(1200)*	1093 *(800)*	2404
Blood sampling and family history questionnaires	1641	1208	2849

Italics = target sample size

Update:

Trial B closed to recruitment in October 2001 with a total of 2215 patients.
Trial A closed at the end of October 2002 with a total of 2236 patients.

ICR-CTSU

Title: TACT: A randomized trial of standard anthracycline-based chemotherapy (fluorouracil, epirubicin and cyclophosphamide [FEC] or epirubicin and CMF [Epi-CMF]) vs FEC followed by sequential docetaxel in women with early breast cancer.
ISRCTN 79718493

Joint Clinical Coordinators:
P. Ellis
Guy's, Kings, St Thomas' Cancer Centre
Medical Oncology research Office
3rd Floor
Thomas Guy House
St Thomas St.
LONDON, SE1 9RT
UNITED KINGDOM
Tel: +44 20 7955 5000
Fax: +44 20 7955 2714
Email: paul.ellis@gstt.sthames.nhs.uk

P. Barrett-Lee
Velindre NHS Trust
WHITCHURCH
CARDIFF, CF14 2TL
UNITED KINGDOM
Tel: +44 02920 316 914
Fax: +44 02920 316 267
Email: peter.barrett-lee@velindre-tr.wales.nhs.uk

Trial Coordinator:
L. Johnson
Clinical Trials & Statistics Unit (ICR-CTSU)
Section of Epidemiology
Institute of Cancer Research
Brookes Lawley Building
Cotswold Road
SUTTON
SURREY, SM2 5NG
UNITED KINGDOM
Tel: +44 20 8722 4188
Fax: +44 20 8770 7876
Email: lindsay.johnson@icr.ac.uk

Summary:
- Opened February 2001
- Target accrual: 3340 – increased to 4000 in January 2003.

Scheme:

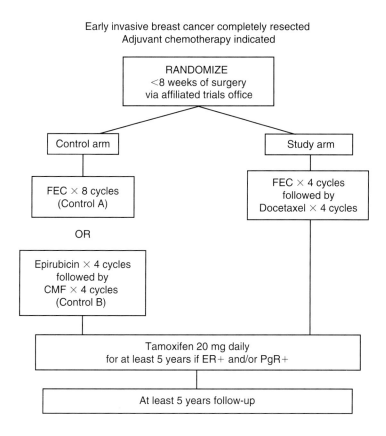

Early invasive breast cancer completely resected
Adjuvant chemotherapy indicated

RANDOMIZE
<8 weeks of surgery
via affiliated trials office

Control arm

Study arm

FEC × 8 cycles
(Control A)

FEC × 4 cycles
followed by
Docetaxel × 4 cycles

OR

Epirubicin × 4 cycles
followed by
CMF × 4 cycles
(Control B)

Tamoxifen 20 mg daily
for at least 5 years if ER+ and/or PgR+

At least 5 years follow-up

Update:

4159 patients entered as of June 2003.

IKA

STUDIES

IKA

Title: Adjuvant chemotherapy with CMF vs observation of premenopausal patients with lymph node-negative but morphometrically unfavourable (Mitotic Activity Index > 10) breast cancer.
(PREMIS = Premenopausal Intervention Study)

Coordinators: J.P.A. Baak
IKA
Plesmanlaan 125
NL-1066 CX AMSTERDAM
THE NETHERLANDS
Tel: +31 20 346 25 30
Fax: +31 20 346 25 25

J. Benraadt
IKA
Plesmanlaan 125
NL-1066 CX AMSTERDAM
THE NETHERLANDS
Tel: +31 20 346 2530
Fax: +31 20 346 2525

Summary:
- Closed in July 1998 (opened in 1990)
- Target accrual: 332 patients

Objective:

To evaluate if adjuvant CMF is beneficial for premenopausal women with operable primary breast cancer without nodal involvement but with otherwise morphometrically unfavourable characteristics.

Scheme:

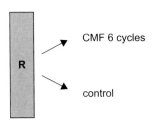

R → CMF 6 cycles

R → control

Update:

Study closed for randomization in July 1998.
280 patients randomized.

Title: Adjuvant treatment with tamoxifen vs nil in postmenopausal women with stage I–III breast cancer.

Coordinator: J.B. Vermorken
IKA
Plesmanlaan 125
NL-1066 CX AMSTERDAM
THE NETHERLANDS
Tel: +31 20 346 2530
Fax: +31 20 346 2525

Summary:
- Study closed in July 1998 (opened in 1982)
- Target accrual: 1230 patients

Scheme:

node-negative / node-positive patients until 1988

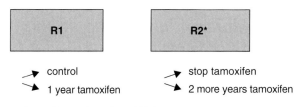

node-positive patients form 1988

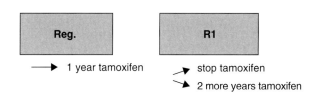

* R2 only for patients on tamoxifen after R1

Update:

Study closed for randomization in January 1994.
1662 patients entered.

IKA

Title: Adjuvant tamoxifen plus combination chemotherapy with Epirubicin and cyclophosphamide vs tamoxifen alone in postmenopausal node-positive breast cancer patients.

Coordinators: J.B. Vermorken
IKA
Plesmanlaan 125
NL-1066 CX AMSTERDAM
THE NETHERLANDS
Tel: +31 20 3462 544
Fax: +31 20 3462 525

J.V.R. Nortier
Leids Universitair Medisch Centrum (LUMC)
Clinical Oncology
Postbus 9600
NL-2300 RC LEIDEN
THE NETHERLANDS
Tel: +31 71 526 3486
Fax: +31 71 526 6760
Email: j.v.r.nortier@lumc.nl

Summary:
- Closed in June 1998 (opened in 1992)
- Target accrual: 500 patients

Objective:

To evaluate the additional effect of "optimal chemotherapy" to tamoxifen in postmenopausal women with node-positive breast cancer, in terms of recurrence rate, disease-free and overall survival.

Scheme:

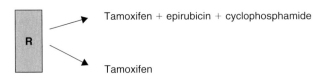

R → Tamoxifen + epirubicin + cyclophosphamide

R → Tamoxifen

Update:

Study closed for randomization in July 1998.
102 patients randomized.

Title: An international randomized trial in Locally Advanced Breast Cancer comparing 6 courses of neo-adjuvant doxorubicin and cyclophosphamide plus GM-CSF or G-CSF with a split course administration of 3 neo-adjuvant and 3 adjuvant cycles including either GM-CSF or G-CSF.
SPINOZA

Coordinators: Dr E. van der Wall
VU Medisch Centrum (VUMC)
Medical Oncology
P.O. Box 7057
NL-1007 MB AMSTERDAM
THE NETHERLANDS
Tel: +31 20 4444 300
Fax: +31 20 4444 355
Email: e.vanderwall@vumc.nl

Dr N. Castaneda
Instituto Nacional de Cancerlogia
Av. San Fernando #22
1400 MEXICO D.F.
MEXICO

Summary:
- Open November 1998
- Target accrual: 600 patients

Objectives:

- To determine the impact of 6 neo-adjuvant cycles of Adriamycin + cyclophosphamide (AC) cycles in comparison with 3 neo-adjuvant cycles on the 3 year disease free survival (DFS) and overall survival of patients with locally advanced breast cancer (LABC), stage IIB, IIIA and IIIB;
- To assess the effect of 6 neo-adjuvant cycles on the clinical and pathological response in comparison with 3 neo-adjuvant cycles;
- To study the effect of GM-CSF on the DFS, clinical and pathological response in comparison with G-CSF;
- To assess the local relapse rate of the two treatment schedules.

Scheme:

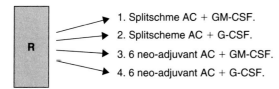

R
1. Splitschme AC + GM-CSF.
2. Splitscheme AC + G-CSF.
3. 6 neo-adjuvant AC + GM-CSF.
4. 6 neo-adjuvant AC + G-CSF.

Update:

Study closed 1 June 2002.
82 patients randomized.

JBCSG

STUDY

JBCSG

Title: Phase II neoadjuvant trial looking at the efficacy of CEF followed by docetaxel for primary breast cancer patients.

Coordinator: M.Toi
Tokyo Medical Center for Cancer and Infectious Diseases
Komagome Hospital
3-18-22, Honkomagome, Bunkyo-ku
TOKYO 113-8677
JAPAN
Tel: +81 3 3823 2101
Fax: +81 3 3824 1552
Email: maktoi77@wa2.so-net.ne.jp

Summary:
- Opened in July 2002
- Target accrual: 100 patients

Objectives:

Primary:
Clinical response, pathological response.

Secondary:
Molecular changes in apoptosis-related molecules, drug-resistance related molecules.

Scheme: *Regimen:*

CEF (500 mg/m^2, 100 mg/m^2) q3 $\times$ 4 cycles $\rightarrow$ docetaxel (75 mg/m2) q3 $\times$ 4 cycles

Update:

Accrual will end in 2003; study will form the basis for larger, multi-centre international trials.

NCIC CTG

STUDIES

NCIC CTG

Title: Double-blind randomized trial of tamoxifen vs placebo in patients with node-positive or high-risk node-negative (tumor $\geq$ 1 cm and either higher histological grade (poorly differentiated, or SBR grade III or MSBR grade V) or lymphatic / vascular invasion or both) breast cancer who have completed CMF, CEF or AC adjuvant chemotherapy.
NCIC CTG Trial MA.12

Chair: V. Bramwell
London Regional Cancer Centre
790 Commissioners Road East
LONDON, ONTARIO N6A 4L6
CANADA
Tel: +1 519 685 8640, ext. 3292
Fax: +1 519 685 8624

Coordinator: B. Graham
NCIC CTG
Queen's University
82-84 Barrie St.
KINGSTON, ONTARIO K7L 3N6
CANADA
Tel: +1 613 533 6430
Fax: +1 613 533 2941

Summary:
- Opened in July 1993
- Target accrual: 800 patients

Objectives:

- To compare the duration of overall survival among premenopausal women with axillary node-positive or high-risk node-negative breast cancer following CEF, or AC chemotherapy who will receive either tamoxifen 20 mg a day for 5 years or placebo. An additional endpoint will be disease-free survival;
- To evaluate the toxicity in patients receiving tamoxifen compared to placebo;
- To monitor FSH, LH and estradiol levels and determine if OS or DFS is affected by hormonal or menopausal status during or at completion of chemotherapy or during or after tamoxifen or placebo treatment.

Scheme:

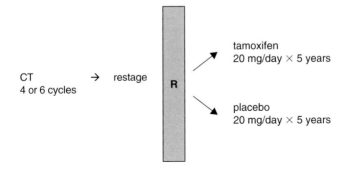

CT → restage **R** tamoxifen 20 mg/day × 5 years

placebo 20 mg/day × 5 years

CT
4 or 6 cycles

Update:

This trial was closed to accrual April 2000.
672 patients were randomized.
Follow-up is ongoing and the analysis is anticipated in 2005.

NCIC CTG

Title: A randomized trial of antiestrogen therapy vs combined antiestrogen and octreotide LAR therapy in the adjuvant treatment of breast cancer in post-menopausal women.
NCIC CTG Trial MA.14

Chair: M. Pollak
Medical Oncology
Sir Mortimer B. Davis
Jewish General Hospital
3755 Chemin de la Côte-Ste-Catherine
MONTREAL, QUEBEC H3T 1E2
CANADA
Tel: +1 514 340 8222, ext. 5530
Fax: +1 514 340 8302

Coordinator: P. Richardson
NCIC CTG
Queen's University
82-84 Barrie St.
KINGSTON, ONTARIO K7L 3N6
CANADA
Tel: +1 613 533 6430
Fax: +1 613 533 2941

Summary:
- Opened in September 1996
- Target accrual: 850 patients

Objectives:

- To compare event-free, recurrence-free and overall survival;
- To compare the two treatment arms with respect to treatment toxicity and quality of life;
- To compare the two treatment arms with respect to effects of treatment on insulin-like growth factor physiology, and to study relationships between insulin-like growth factor physiology and outcome.

Scheme:

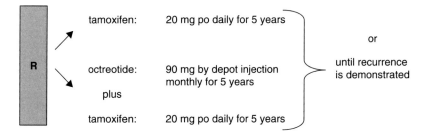

Update:

This trial was closed to accrual in July 2001.
667 patients were randomized.
Analysis is anticipated for 2005.

NCIC CTG

Title: A phase III randomized double blind study of letrozole vs placebo in women with primary breast cancer completing five or more years of adjuvant tamoxifen.
BIG 01-97 / NCIC CTG MA.17

Chair: P. Goss
The Toronto Hospital
(General Division)
200 Elizabeth St.
M/LW 2-018
TORONTO, ONTARIO M5G 2C4
CANADA
Tel: +1 416 946 4534
Fax: +1 416 946 2983
Email: pegoss@interlog.com

Coordinators: M. Palmer and C. Elliott
NCIC CTG
Queen's University
82-84 Barrie St.
KINGSTON, ONTARIO K7L 3N6
CANADA
Tel: +1 613 533 6430
Fax: +1 613 533 2941

Summary:
- Opened in August 1998
- Target accrual: 4800 patients

Objectives:

- To compare disease-free survival and overall survival;
- To compare incidence of contralateral breast cancer, and long-term clinical and laboratory safety;
- To evaluate quality of life.

Scheme:

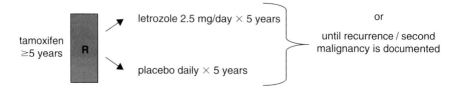

Update:

This study exceeded its accrual goal and closed in May 2002.
5187 patients were randomized.
The first interim analysis is anticipated in Summer 2004.

Title: *NCIC CTG MA.17 Companion study (2):* The influence of letrozole on bone mineral density in women with primary breast cancer completing five or more years of adjuvant tamoxifen.
BIG 01-97 / NCIC MA.17B

Chair: P. Goss
The Toronto Hospital
(General Division)
200 Elizabeth St.
M/LW 2-018
TORONTO, ONTARIO M5G 2C4
CANADA
Tel: +1 416 946 4534
Fax: +1 416 946 2983
Email: pegoss@interlog.com

Coordinators: M. Palmer and C. Elliott
NCIC CTG
Queen's University
82-84 Barrie St.
KINGSTON, ONTARIO K7L 3N6
CANADA
Tel: +1 613 533 6430
Fax: +1 613 533 2941

Summary:
- Opened in Fall 1999
- Target accrual: 200 patients

Endpoints:

- Percentage change in BMD from baseline in the L2–L4 (PA) region of the spine and hip at 2 years and 5 years;
- Proportion of women who develop BMD below the absolute threshold for osteoporosis;
- Percentage change in bone biomarkers from baseline;
- Clinical safety of letrozole with respect to osteoporosis in the evaluation of fractures (collected as part of the core protocol).

Scheme:

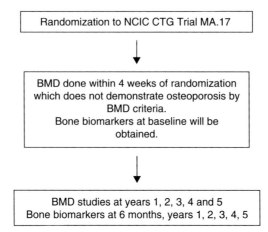

Update:

The trial closed in August 2002 with 226 patients accrued.
The first 2 year analysis is planned for the summer of 2004.

Title: *NCIC CTG MA.17 Companion study (1):* The influence of letrozole on serum lipid concentrations in women with primary breast cancer who have completed five years of adjuvant tamoxifen.
BIG 01-97 / NCIC CTG MA.17L

Chair: P. Goss
The Toronto Hospital
(General Division)
200 Elizabeth St.
M/LW 2-018
TORONTO, ONTARIO M5G 2C4
CANADA
Tel: +1 416 946 4534
Fax: +1 416 946 2983
Email: pegoss@interlog.com

Coordinators: M. Palmer and C. Elliott
NCIC CTG
Queen's University
82-84 Barrie St.
KINGSTON, ONTARIO K7L 3N6
CANADA
Tel: +1 613 533 6430
Fax: +1 613 533 2941

Summary:
- Opened in August 1999
- Target accrual: 300 patients

Objective:

To evaluate the effects of letrozole on serum lipid parameters in postmenopausal women treated with letrozole or placebo following at least five years of adjuvant tomoxifen therapy for breast cancer.

Primary:
- Mean % change from baseline in LDL cholesterol.
- Mean % change from baseline in total cholesterol.

Secondary:
- Incidence of clinically relevant changes in lipid parameters.
- Incidence of requirement for prescribing of antilipidemic medication and/or diet change.

Scheme:

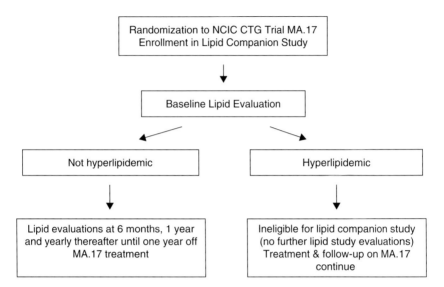

Update:

This study reached its accrual goal of 347 patients and closed in May 2002.
The first analysis at 2 years is anticipated for the summer of 2004.

Title: A phase III study of regional radiation therapy in early breast cancer.
             NCIC CTG Trial MA.20

Chair: T. Whelan
             Hamilton Regional Cancer Centre
             699 Concession St.
             HAMILTON, ONTARIO L8V 5C2
             CANADA
             Tel: +1 905 387 9711, ext. 64501
             Fax: +1 905 575 6308

Coordinator: C. Savage
             NCIC CTG
             Queen's University
             82-84 Barrie St.
             KINGSTON, ONTARIO K7L 3N6
             CANADA
             Tel: +1 613 533 6430
             Fax: +1 613 533 2941

Summary:
- Ready to open
- Target accrual: 1822 patients

Objectives:

- To improve the outcome of women with early breast cancer treated with breast conserving therapy – BCT (lumpectomy and breast irradiation) – and adjuvant systemic therapy – AST (chemotherapy and/or hormonal therapy);
- To determine if regional radiation therapy (to the ipsilateral supraclavicular, axillary and internal mammary nodes) in addition to breast irradiation prolongs survival in women with early breast cancer compared with breast irradiation alone;
- To compare disease-free survival in these two treatment approaches;
- To compare isolated local regional disease-free survival in these two treatment approaches;
- To compare distant disease-free survival in these two treatment approaches;
- To evaluate the toxicity effects of these two treatment approaches;
- To evaluate the quality of life associated with these two treatment approaches;
- To determine the cosmetic outcomes of these two treatment approaches.

Scheme:

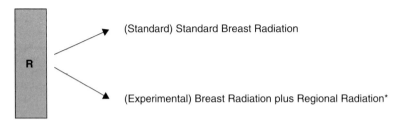

(Standard) Standard Breast Radiation

(Experimental) Breast Radiation plus Regional Radiation*

Radiotherapy must begin within 8 weeks of chemotherapy completion (unless given currently with CMF) or within 16 weeks of the last surgical procedure for patients receiving hormonal therapy only.

* Modified wide tangent technique + supraclavicular and axillary fields

Update:

The study was activated December 1999 and as of February 2003, 568 patients have been accrued.
This trial is now on CTSU menu and has been endorsed by NSABP, SWOG, NCCTG and TROG (Australia).

Title: A phase III adjuvant trial of sequenced EC + GCSF → Taxol vs sequenced AC → Taxol vs CEF as therapy for premenopausal women and early postmenopausal women who have had potentally curative surgery for node positive or high-risk node negative breast cancer.
NCIC CTG Trial MA.21

Chairs: M. Levine
Hamilton Regional Cancer Centre
699 Concession St.
HAMILTON, ONTARIO L8V 5C2
CANADA
Tel: +1 905 387 9711
Fax: +1 905 575 6308

M. Burnell
St Johns Regional Cancer Center
St Johns, NEW BRUNSWICK
CANADA

Coordinator: Sonia Schellenberger
NCIC Clinical Trials Group
Queen's University
82-84 Barrie St.
KINGSTON, ONTARIO K7L 3N6
CANADA
Tel: +1 613 533 6430
Fax: +1 613 533 2941
Email: sschellenberger@ctg.queensu.ca

Summary:
- To be opened Spring 2000
- Target accrual: 1500 patients

Objectives:

- To compare disease-free survival and overall survival among women with high-risk operable breast cancer following surgical resection of all known disease who are randomized to receive as adjuvant therapy either cyclophosphamide, Epirubicin and 5 fluorouracil, (CEF), or Epirubicin and cyclophosphamide with GCSF followed by Taxol (EC + GCSF/T), or adriamycin and cyclophosphamide followed by Taxol (AC/T);
- To compare the rates of toxicities among the patients who receive either CEF, EC + GCSF/T or AC/T;
- To compare the quality of life among patients who receive either CEF, EC + GCSF/T, or AC/T.

Scheme:

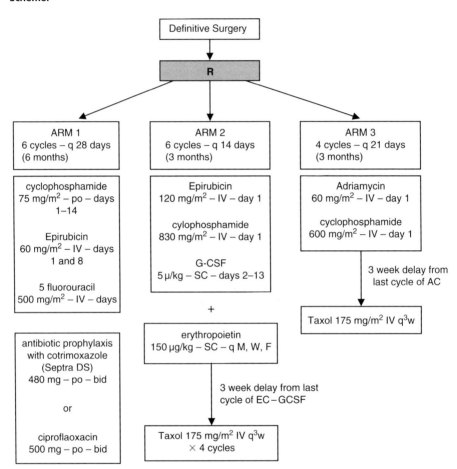

Update:

The study opened in December 2000 and as of February 2003 accrued 774 women. The study is now on the CTSU menu and has been endorsed by SWOG and NCCTG. Many independent centers in the US are also participating.

Title: A randomized phase III trial of exemestane vs anastrozole with or without celecoxib in postmenopausal women with receptor positive primary breast cancer.
NCIC CTG Trial MA.27

Chair: Dr Paul Goss

Coordinator: Catherine Elliot

Summary:
- As of March 2003 the protocol had almost completed its circuit of regulatory approvals and was due to begin accruing April 2003.
- Canadian sites will participate through NCIC CTG in the usual manner; US sites will participate through CTSU, the BMB will not be handling the drug distribution for this trial; the Kingston General Hospital Pharmacy will be distributing drugs to all sites in Canada and the US. For more information visit the NCIC website: address

Primary endpoint:

- Event free survival

Secondary endpoints:

- Overall survival
- Time to distant recurrence
- Incidence of contralateral breast cancer
- Long-term clinical and laboratory safety

Patient population:

Post-menopausal women who have histologically or cytologically confirmed, receptor-positive, adequately excised, primary breast cancer.

Stratification:

Parameters include lymph node status (negative, positive or unknown), prior adjuvant chemotherapy (yes, no), current use of low dose prophylactic aspirin of $\leqslant 81\,mg/day$ (yes, no).

Objectives:

- To determine the event-free survival (EFS) between women treated with exemestane or anastrozole as adjuvant therapy;
- To determine the effect on EFS of adding celecoxib to an aromatase inhibitor;
- To compare fracture incidence, cardiovascular morbidity and mortality and overall toxicities in the four treatment groups.

Scheme:

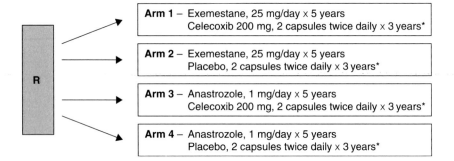

Treatment is for 5 years or until recurrence / second malignancy is documented.

* Celecoxib / Placebo component is blinded

NNBC-3

STUDY

NNBC-3

Title: Randomized study comparing 6 × FEC with 3 × FEC followed by 3 × docetaxel in high-risk node-negative patients with operable breast cancer: Comparison of efficacy and evaluation of clinico-pathological and biochemical markers as risk selection criteria.

Coordinator: Prof Dr med Christoph Thomssen (PI)
Klinik und Poliklinik fuer Frauenheilkunde und Geburtshilfe
Universitaetsklinikum Eppendorf
University of Hamburg
Martinistr. 52
D-20246 HAMBURG
GERMANY
Tel: +49 40 42803 8172 / 3510
Fax: +49 40 42803 2511
Email: oben@uke.uni-hamburg.de

Summary:
- Opened in November 2002
- Target accrual: 5700 patients (2572 in the high risk group to randomize)

Objectives:

- To investigate whether substituting the last 3 cycles of a standard adjuvant $FE_{100}C$ by 3 cycles of docetaxel could improve the disease-free survival of high-risk node-negative breast cancer patients;
- To compare the risk assessment by clinico-pathological characteristics with the risk assessment by the invasion markers uPA/PAI-1;
- To investigate whether registered patients can still be discriminated with respect to their risk of first recurrence and survival when the other selection criterion is used;
- To investigate prospectively whether patients with HER-2/neu overexpression have a higher benefit by an anthracycline-taxane sequence than by an anthracycline combination alone.

Scheme:

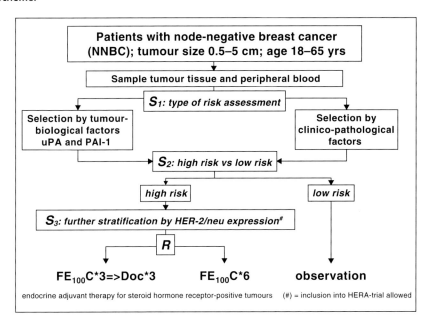

Patients with node-negative breast cancer (NNBC); tumour size 0.5–5 cm; age 18–65 yrs

Sample tumour tissue and peripheral blood

S_1: type of risk assessment

Selection by tumour-biological factors uPA and PAI-1

Selection by clinico-pathological factors

S_2: high risk vs low risk

high risk

low risk

S_3: further stratification by HER-2/neu expression[#]

R

$FE_{100}C*3 => Doc*3$

$FE_{100}C*6$

observation

endocrine adjuvant therapy for steroid hormone receptor-positive tumours   (#) = inclusion into HERA-trial allowed

Update:

25 patients entered so far (2 centres opened as of March 2003).

NWAST

STUDY

NWAST

Title: Adjuvant chemotherapy with or without intensification with hematopoietic stem cell support in patients with stage II or III breast cancer, involving ≥ 4 axillary lymph nodes.

Coordinators: S. Rodenhuis
The Netherlands Cancer Institute
Antoni van Leeuwenhoekhuis
Dept of Medical Oncology
Plesmanlaan 121
NL-1066 CX AMSTERDAM
THE NETHERLANDS
Tel: +31 20 512 2870
Fax: +31 20 617 2572

E.G.E. de Vries
University Hospital Groningen
Dept Internal Medicine
Division of Medical Oncology
P.O. Box 30001
NL-9700 RB GRONINGEN
THE NETHERLANDS
Tel: +31 50 361 61 61
Fax: +31 50 361 48 62

Summary:
- Closed in June 1999 (opened in 1993)
- Target accrual : 880 patients

Objectives:

- To determine whether very-high-dose chemotherapy with autologous stem cell support should be offered to relatively young patients with high-risk breast cancer as part of adjuvant therapy;
- To compare the toxicity of a standard anthracycline-based adjuvant chemotherapy consisting of five courses of FEC with 4 courses of FEC followed by very-high-dose chemotherapy;
- The design of the study will allow the evaluation of the potential survival benefit of chemotherapy intensification with autologous hematopoietic stem cell support as a method of preventing relapse. It will also serve to determine their relative costs of these treatment strategies; a cost-effectiveness study will be performed in parallel.

Scheme:

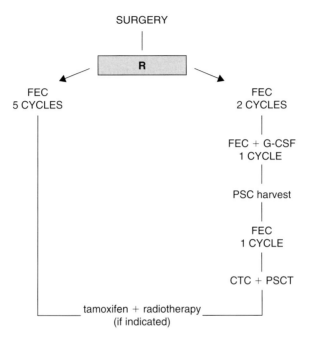

SURGERY

R

FEC
5 CYCLES

FEC
2 CYCLES

FEC + G-CSF
1 CYCLE

PSC harvest

FEC
1 CYCLE

CTC + PSCT

tamoxifen + radiotherapy
(if indicated)

Total dose: CTC = cyclophosphamide 6000 mg/m^2, thiotepa 480 mg/m^2, carboplatin 1600 mg/m^2
FEC = cyclophosphamide 500 mg/m^2, epidoxorubicin 90 mg/m^2, 5-fluorouracil 500 mg/m^2

Update:

Study closed in June 1999.
885 patients randomized.

PEGASE

STUDY

PEGASE

Title: Prospective phase III trial comparing sequential high-dose chemotherapy to conventional FEC100 regimen for high-risk breast cancer patients.
PEGASE 06

Coordinator: Pr P. Pouillart
Institut Curie
26, rue d'Ulm
75 231 PARIS cedex 05
FRANCE
Tel: +33 (0)1 44 32 40 00 – +33 (0)4 91 22 36 01
Fax: +33 (0)1 44 32 41 19 – +33 (0)4 91 22 36 01

Summary:
- Opened January 2001
- Target accrual: 400 patients

Objective:

15% increase in DFS at 3 years

Scheme: For N > 7, less than 60 y, non metastatic unilateral breast tumor either 6 FEC100 or 4 cycles epirubicin 150 mg/m^2, cyclophosphamide 4 g/m^2 every 3 weeks with PBCP rescue after cycles 2, 3, 4.
Tamoxifen if ER or PR+.

Update:

91 inclusions as of March 2003.

Title: Phase III trial testing adjuvant chemotherapy for inflammatory breast cancer patients treated with sequential high-dose chemotherapy as neo-adjuvant treatment.
PEGASE 07

Coordinator: Pr P. Viens
Institut Paoli-Calmettes
232, boulevard Ste Marguerite
13 273 MARSEILLE cedex 09
FRANCE
Tel: +33 (0)4 91 22 35 37
Fax: +33 (0)4 91 22 36 01

Summary:
- Opened December 2000
- Target accrual: 176 patients

Objective:

20% gain for event free survival

Scheme: Induction arm with 4 cycles of epirubicin 150 mg/m^2, cyclophosphamide 4 g/m2 every 3 weeks with PBCP rescue after cycles 2, 3, 4 then surgery. Randomization after surgery between nothing or 4 cycles of Taxotere 85 mg/m^2, 5FU 750 mg/m^2/d continuous infusion over 5 days every 3 weeks. Tamoxifen if ER or PR+.

Update:

87 inclusions as of March 2003.

SBG

STUDIES

SBG

Title: High-dose chemotherapy + autologous stem cell transplantation compared with dose escalating chemotherapy in breast cancer with poor prognosis ⩾ 8 positive lymph nodes or ⩾ 5 lymph nodes combined with R-combined with either G II–III or high S-phase.
A randomized study.
SBG 9401

Coordinators: J. Bergh
Radiumhemmet
Karolinska Institute & Hospital
S-17176 STOCKHOLM
SWEDEN
Tel: +46 8 51 77 62 79
Fax: +46 8 51 77 51 96
Email: jonas.bergh@ks.se

N. Wilking
Dept of Oncology
Karolinska Sjukhuset
S-10401 STOCKHOLM
SWEDEN
Tel: +46 87 29 43 09
Fax: +46 87 29 51 96

Summary:
- Closed in March 1998 (opened 1 March 1994)
- Target accrual: 500 patients

Objectives:

- To compare disease-free survival of high-risk breast cancer patients treated with either high-dose chemotherapy + autologous stem cell transplantation or dose-escalated chemotherapy (CEC) both as adjuvant treatment;
- To compare survival, safety, dose-intensity and total dose between the two treatment arms;
- To assess quality of life.

Scheme:

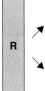

R

Arm A
dose-escalating FEC + filgrastim → tamoxifen for 5 years + RT
9 cycles

Arm B
FEC 3 cycles + filgrastim (cycle 3) → high-dose chemotherapy + PBPC support → tamoxifen for 5 years + RT

Arm A:

Dose escalating FEC
I step: 5 FU 600 mg/m^2 Epirubicin 75 mg/m^2, cyclo 900 mg/m^2
II step: 5 FU 600 mg/m^2, Epirubicin 90 mg/m^2, cyclo 1200 mg/m^2
III step: 5 FU 600 mg/m^2, Epirubicin 105 mg/m^2, cyclo 1500 mg/m^2
IV step: 5 FU 600 mg/m^2, Epirubicin 120 mg/m^2, cyclo 1800 mg/m^2

Arm B:

Induction FEC
Cycles 1–2: 5 FU 600 mg/m^2, Epirubicin 60 mg/m^2, cyclo 600 mg/m^2
Cycle 3:   5 FU 600 mg/m^2, Epirubicin 60 mg/m^2, cyclo 1200 mg/m^2 + G-CSF

High-dose CT:

Cycle 4: (cyclophosphamide 1.5 g/m^2 + thiotepa 125 mg/m^2 + carboplatin 200 mg/m^2) days -7 to -4

Update:

Study closed March 1998.
525 patients randomized.
Reported in *The Lancet* 2000.
New update ongoing.

SBG

Title: Standard CEF-60 vs tailored CEF in high-risk primary breast cancer.
SBG CEF-60

Chair: C. Blomquist
Dept of Oncology
Uppsala University
SE-75185 UPPSALA
SWEDEN
Tel: +35 840 548 6580
Email: carl.blomquist@onkologi.uu.sv

Summary: • Target accrual = 1500
• Opened 2001

Scheme: First cycle of CEF-60:
• If WBG GR III/IV: continue with 6 cycles of CEF-60/ reduced dose
• If WBG GR 0–II: randomize to 6 cycles of CEF-60/ escalated CEF

Update:

Accrual as of March 2003: 1100.

Title: HABITS – Hormonal replacement therapy after breast cancer diagnosis – is it safe?
BIG 03-97

Principal Investigator: L. Holmberg
Regional Oncologic Center
University Hospital
S-75185 UPPSALA
SWEDEN
Tel: +46 18 15 19 10
Fax: +46 18 17 44 14
Email: lars.holmberg@roc.lul.se

Summary: • Opened in 1998
• Target accrual: 1300 patients

Objectives:

• To investigate in women with radically treated in situ, stage I or early stage II breast cancer if the use of hormone replacement therapy (HRT for menopausal symptoms) is safe concerning risk of breast cancer recurrence;
• To look at quality of life and risk of breast cancer death.

Scheme:

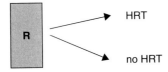

R → HRT

R → no HRT

Update:

431 patients entered as of February 2003.

WMBG

STUDIES

WMBG

Title: aTTom – adjuvant Tamoxifen Treatment – offer more?

Coordinator: Dr Philip Perry
Cancer Research UK Clinical Trials Unit
Institute for Cancer Studies
The University of Birmingham
EDGBASTON
BIRMINGHAM, B15 2TT
UNITED KINGDOM
Tel: +44 121 414 7626
Fax: +44 121 414 3700
Email: aTTom@bham.ac.uk

Summary: *Objective:*

A large, uniquely simple, randomized study to assess much more reliably the balance of benefits and risks of prolonging adjuvant tamoxifen treatment in early breast cancer. Eligibility criteria are pragmatic, with randomization taking place at the point when *substantial uncertainty* arises as to whether to stop or to continue tamoxifen.

Target Accrual: 8000 patients from the UK and Republic of Ireland; 20,000 patients worldwide, in collaboration with its global counterpart ATLAS (Adjuvant Tamoxifen – Longer Against Shorter), which is coordinated by the Clinical Trial Service Unit at the University of Oxford, UK.

Scheme:

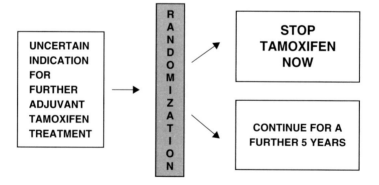

Update:

A total of 6890 patients had been randomized into aTTom by end of June 2003. The best ever monthly recruitment was recorded in January 2003, with 118 patients randomized. It is projected that the target of 8000 patients will be reached in mid-2004. A total of 11785 patients had been randomized into ATLAS by July 2003.

WMBG

Title: Sequencing of Chemotherapy and Radiotherapy in Adjuvant Breast cancer.
SECRAB

Coordinator: Dr Sarah Bowden
Cancer Research UK Clinical Trials Unit
Institute for Cancer Studies
The University of Birmingham
Vincent Drive
EDGBASTON
BIRMINGHAM, B15 2TT
UNITED KINGDOM
Tel: +44 (0) 121 414 4371
Fax: +44 (0) 121 414 3700
Email: BTT@bham.ac.uk

Summary: *Objective:*

To determine if local control can be improved by the synchronous delivery of adjuvant chemotherapy and radiotherapy, thereby not delaying the administration of either modality; and to determine if the two treatment modalities can be given together safely.

Target Accrual: 2250 patients

Scheme:

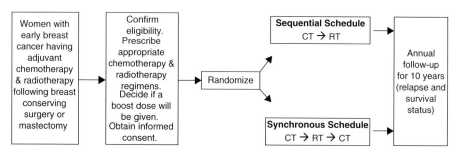

Update:

The study opened for recruitment in July 1998. On the first of July 2003 1957 patients had been randomized by 58 consultants from 42 centres with in the UK. Recruitment is currently averaging 25 patients per month and at this rate of accrual we should reach our recruitment target of 2250 patients in June 2004. The study will, however, close to recruitment in March 2004.

Title: A phase III randomized trial of gemcitabine in paclitaxel-containing, epirubicin-based, adjuvant chemotherapy for women with early stage breast cancer.
tAnGo

Coordinator: Dr Helen Howard
Cancer Research UK Clinical Trials Unit
Institute for Cancer Studies
The University of Birmingham
EDGBASTON
BIRMINGHAM, B15 2TT
UNITED KINGDOM
Tel: +44 121 414 3017
Fax: +44 121 414 3700
Email: tango@trials.bham.ac.uk

Summary: *Objective:*

To determine whether the addition of gemcitabine to the second phase of a control regimen of epirubicin and cyclophosphamide followed by paclitaxel improves disease-free survival in relation to epirubicin and cyclophosphamide followed by paclitaxel alone, in women presenting with early stage breast cancer.

Target Accrual: 3000 patients

Scheme:

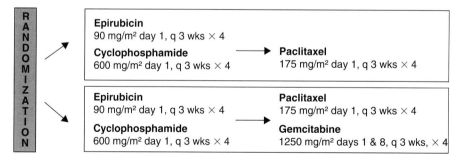

R
A
N
D
O
M
I
Z
A
T
I
O
N

Epirubicin
90 mg/m² day 1, q 3 wks × 4
Cyclophosphamide
600 mg/m² day 1, q 3 wks × 4
→ Paclitaxel
175 mg/m² day 1, q 3 wks × 4

Epirubicin
90 mg/m² day 1, q 3 wks × 4
Cyclophosphamide
600 mg/m² day 1, q 3 wks × 4
→ Paclitaxel
175 mg/m² day 1, q 3 wks × 4
Gemcitabine
1250 mg/m² days 1 & 8, q 3 wks, × 4

Update:

Recruitment commenced in November 2001 with a preliminary safety study which was mandatory for the first 130 patients enrolled. This involved detailed monitoring of patients' cardiac and pulmonary function. Accrual of this substudy was completed in October 2002 and the main trial was officially launched in January 2003. As of end of June 2003, a total of 386 patients have been enrolled on the study from 40 UK centres. Approximately 65 further UK centres have expressed interest in participating in the study.

Title: *Tamoxifen* and *Exemestane* *Adjuvant* *Multicentre* Trial
            TEAM

Coordinator: Dr Margaret Grant
            Cancer Research UK Clinical Trials Unit
            Institute for Cancer Studies
            The University of Birmingham
            EDGBASTON
            BIRMINGHAM, B15 2TT
            UNITED KINGDOM
            Tel: +44 121 414 3797
            Fax: +44 121 414 3700
            Email: team@trials.bham.ac.uk

Summary: *Objective:*

            To compare the use of tamoxifen, a standard adjuvant hormone therapy,
            with exemestane, an aromatase inhibitor, in the adjuvant treatment of
            postmenopausal women with early stage breast cancer. Quality of life,
            pathology and bone substudies are included as part of the British arm
            of the trial.

Target Accrual: 5200 patients worldwide, with 740 from the UK/RoI.

Scheme:

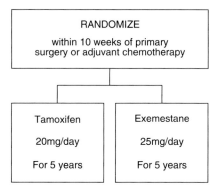

Update:

The first patient was randomized in December 2001. As of May 2003, 658 patients were
recruited from 95 participating centres. The main UK arm of the trial is now closed,
however, accrual into the bone sub-study continues. It is estimated that the trial will reach
its full accrual target by October 2003.

WSG

STUDIES

WSG

Title: WSG and AGO-Mamma Intergroup Study:
Randomized phase III trial of EC → Doc: adjuvant chemotherapy of
breast carcinoma with 1-3 positive lymph nodes.
AM02

Chairs: U. Nitz (WSG)
Dept of Gynecology
University of Düsseldorf
DÜSSELDORF
GERMANY
Tel: +49 21 1811 7550
Fax: +49 21 1312 283
Email: nitzu@uni-duesseldorf.de
Website: www.brustcentrum.de

W. Kuhn (AGO-Mamma)
Dept of Gynecology
University of Bonn
Sigmund-Freudstr. 25
53105 BONN
GERMANY

Biostatistics Unit: H.-P. Adams
Dr Horst-Schmid-Kliniken
Klinik für Gynäkologie
Ludwig-Erhardstr. 100
65199 BONN
GERMANY

Summary:
- Opened in September 2000
- Target accrual: 2000

Objective:

Event free survival (EFS) and overall survival (OS).
Comparison of: a) Toxicity
                b) Quality of Life (QOL)
                c) Cost effectiveness analysis

Scheme:

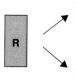

4 × cyclophosphamide / epirubicin (EC, 90/600 mg/m^2) →
4 × docetaxel (T, 100mg/m^2) 3-weekly

6 × cyclophosphamide / methotrexate / 5-fluoruracil (CMF, 600t/40/600 mg/m^2, day 1+8, 4-weekly

OR

6 × cylcophosphamide / 5-fluoruracil / epirubicin (FEC, 500, 100, 500 mg/m^2)

Update:

890 patients entered as of early July 2003.

WSG

Title: WSG Study: Randomized phase III trial of adjuvant CEF/TAC
chemotherapy +/− Darbepoetin alfa for patients with primary breast
cancer and more than 3 positive axillary lymph nodes.
ARA 3-Study / AM03

Chair: U. Nitz (WSG)
Dept of Gynecology
University of Düsseldorf
DÜSSELDORF
GERMANY
Tel: +49 21 1811 7550
Fax: +49 21 1312 283
Email: nitzu@uni-duesseldorf.de
Website: www.brustcentrum.de

Biostatistics Unit: K. Ulm
Klinikum rechts der Isar
Institut für Medizinische Statistik und Epidemiologie
Ismaningerstr. 22
81675 MÜNCHEN
GERMANY

Summary:
- Opening in August 2003
- Target accrual: 1000

Objectives:

- Event free survival (EFS)
- Overall Survival (OS)
- Comparison of toxicity, anaemia and cognitive function
- Comparison of fatigue syndrome.

Scheme:

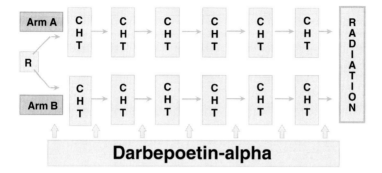

CHT: **TAC:** 6 × docetaxel 75 mg/m^2 + doxorubicin 50mg/m^2 + cyclophosphamide 500 mg/m^2 q3w
or **CEF:** 6 × cyclophosphamide 500 mg/m^2 plus epirubicin 100 mg/m^2 plus 5-FU 500 mg/m^2 q3w

R = randomization

Update:

Study will start in August 2003.

YBCRG

STUDY

YBCRG

Title: Does *A*djuvant *Z*oledronic acid red*U*ce *RE*currence in patients with high risk localised breast cancer? – The AZURE Trial

Coordinator: Miss Liz Graham
Senior Trial Co-ordinator
Northern and Yorkshire Clinical Trials and Research Unit
17 Springfield Mount
LEEDS, LS2 9NG
WEST YORKSHIRE
ENGLAND
Tel: +0113 343 1498
Fax: +0113 343 1471
Email: medehg@leeds.ac.uk

Summary:
- Due to open to recruitment in August 2003
- Target accrual: 3300 patients

Objective:

It is the aim of this prospective, randomized, open label, parallel group trial to determine whether adjuvant treatment with 4 mg zoledronic acid with (neo)adjuvant chemotherapy and/or adjuvant hormonal therapy is superior to (neo)adjuvant chemotherapy and/or adjuvant hormonal therapy alone in improving the disease-free and bone metastasis-free survival of stage II/III breast cancer patients.

Scheme:

Patients will be randomly allocated to receive either zoledronic acid or allocation to a control group.

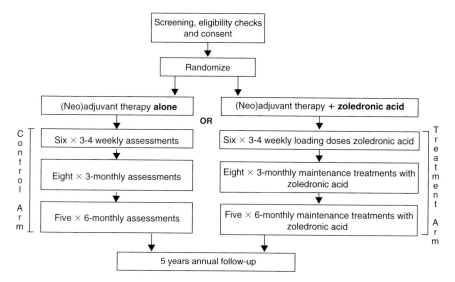

Update:

It is hoped that recruitment will commence in August 2003 and that participation in the trial will involve centres nationally and internationally.

U.S. INTERGROUP

U.S. INTERGROUP CONTACT DETAILS

Group:	American College of Surgeons Oncology Group **(ACOSOG)**
Chair:	Samuel A. Wells, Jr, MD DUMC Box 3627 DURHAM, NC 27710 USA Tel: +1 919 668 8435 Fax: +1 919 668 7123 Email: wells029@surgerytrials.duke.edu
Administrator:	Nancy Jenkins DUMC Box 3627 DURHAM, NC 27710 USA Tel: +1 919 668 8442 Fax: +1 919 668 7122 Email: jenki042@surgerytrials.duke.edu
Group Statistician:	James Herndon, PhD DUMC Box 3627 DURHAM, NC 27710 USA Tel: +1 919 668 8145 Fax: +1 919 668 7122 Email: hernd001@surgerytrials.duke.edu
Administrative/ Statistical Office:	DUMC Box 3627 DURHAM, NC 27710 USA Tel: +1 919 668 8400 Fax: +1 919 668 7122
Courier/Delivery Address:	2400 Pratt St. DURHAM, NC 27705 USA
Website:	www.acosog.org

Group:	Cancer and Leukemia Group B **(CALGB)**
Chair:	Richard L. Schilsky, MD, Chairman
	Central Office of the Chair
	208 South LaSalle St., Suite 2000
	CHICAGO, IL 60604-1104
	USA
	Tel: +1 773 702 9171
	Fax: +1 312 345 0117
	Email: rs27@uchicago.edu
Operations Office:	Jean Roark, Group Administrator
	208 South LaSalle St., Suite 2000
	CHICAGO, IL 60604-1104
	USA
	Tel: +1 773 702 8672
	Fax: +1 312 345 0117
	Email: jroark@uchicago.edu
Statistical Office:	Stephen L. George, PhD
	Prof of Biostatistics
	Cancer Center Biostatistics
	P.O. Box 3958
	Duke University Medical Center
	DURHAM, NC 27710
	USA
	Tel: +1 919 681 5003
	Fax: +1 919 681 8028
	Email: sgeorge@ccstat.mc.duke.edu
Express Mail to:	Duke University Medical Center
	Cancer Center Biostatistics
	Hanes House
	Room 219
	Trent Drive
	DURHAM, NC 27708
	USA
Website:	www.calgb.org

Group:	Eastern Cooperative Oncology Group **(ECOG)**
Chair:	R.L. Comis ECOG Group Chair's Office 1818 Market St., #1100 PHILADELPHIA, PA 19103-9103 USA Tel: +1 215 789 3645 Fax: +1 267 256 5291 Email: rcomis@ecogchair.org
Director of Operations:	D. Marinucci ECOG Group Chair's Office 1818 Market St., #1100 PHILADELPHIA, PA 19103-9103 USA Tel: +1 215 789 3645 Fax: +1 267 256 5291 Email: dmarinucci@ecogchair.org
Coordinating Center (Operations & Data Management):	S. Hurley ECOG Coordinating Center 900 Commonwealth Avenue BOSTON, MA 02215 USA Tel: +1 617 632 3610 Fax: +1 617 632 5414 Email: hurley.sheilah@jimmy.harvard.edu
Statistical Center:	Robert Gray, PhD Division of Biostatistics and Epidemiology Dana-Farber Cancer Institute Mayer 2A 44 Binney St. BOSTON, MA 02115 USA Tel: +1 617 632 3012 Fax: +1 617 632 2444 Email: gray.robert@jimmy.harvard.edu
Website:	www.ecog.org

Group:	National Surgical Adjuvant Breast and Bowel Project **(NSABP)**

Chair:
N. Wolmark
National Surgical Adjuvant Breast and Bowel Project
East Commons Professional Building
Four Allegheny Center, 5th Floor
PITTSBURGH, PA 15212-5234
USA
Tel: +1 412 330 4600
Fax: +1 412 330 4660
Email: ywolmark@nsabp.org

Assistant to Chair:
K. McCaffrey
National Surgical Adjuvant Breast and Bowel Project
Allegheny General Hospital
Allegheny Cancer Center, 5th Floor
320 E North Avenue
PITTSBURGH, PA 15212-4772
USA
Tel: +1 412 359 8227
Fax: +1 412 359 3096
Email: kmccaffr@wpahs.org

Operations Center:
NSABP Operations Center
East Commons Professional Building
Four Allegheny Center, 5th Floor
PITTSBURGH, PA 15212-5234
USA

**Associate Chair/
Director of Operations:**
D.L. Wickerham
Tel: +1 412 330 4600
Fax: +1 412 330 4660
Email: larry.wickerham@nsabp.org

**Membership
Affairs Section:**
M. Ketner
Tel: +1 412 330 4624
Fax: +1 412 330 4662
Email: mary.ketner@nsabp.org

**Regulatory
Affairs Section:**
J. Mull
Tel: +1 412 330 4625
Fax: +1 412 330 4661
Email: joyce.mull@nsabp.org

Clinical Coordinating Section:	B. Harkins Tel: +1 412 330 4643 Fax: +1 412 330 4660 Email: barbara.harkins@nsabp.org
Public Relations and Communications Section:	L. Garvey Tel: +1 412 330 4621 Fax: +1 412 330 4645 Email: lori.garvey@nsabp.org
Finance and Sponsored Projects Section:	D. Szczepankowski Tel: +1 412 330 4610 Fax: +1 412 330 4260 Email: donnas@nsabp.org
Biostatistical Center:	J. Bryant NSABP Biostatistical Center One Sterling Plaza 201 North Craig St., Suite 500 PITTSBURGH, PA 15213 USA Tel: +1 412 383 2554 Fax: +1 412 383 1387 Email: bryant@nsabp.pitt.edu
Website:	www.nsabp.pitt.edu

Group:	Radiation Therapy Oncology Group **(RTOG)**
Chair:	W.J. Curran, Jr
	Radiation Therapy Oncology Group
	1101 Market St., 14th Floor
	PHILADELPHIA, PA 19107
	USA
	Tel: +1 215 955 6700
	Fax: +1 215 955 0412
	Email: walter.curran@mail.tju.edu
Operations and	T. Wudarski
Statistical Office:	1101 Market St., 14th Floor
	PHILADELPHIA, PA 19107
	USA
	Tel: +1 215 574 3205
	Fax: +1 215 923 1737
	Email: twudarski@phila.acr.org
Website:	www.rtog.org

U.S. INTERGROUP STUDY DETAILS

ACOSOG

Title: A prognostic study of sentinel node and bone marrow micrometastases in women with clinical T1 or T2 N0 M0 breast cancer.
ACOSOG Z0010

Principal investigator: A.E. Giuliano
John Wayne Cancer Institute
2200 Santa Monica Boulevard, Suite 113
SANTA MONICA, CA 90404-2302
USA
Tel: +1 310 829 8089
Fax: +1 310 998 3995

Summary:
- Opened May 10, 1999
- Target accrual: 5300 eligible and evaluable patients

Objectives:

- To estimate the prevalence and to evaluate the prognostic significance of sentinel node micrometastases detected by IHC;
- To estimate the prevalence and to evaluate the prognostic significance of bone marrow micrometastases detected by ICC;
- To evaluate the hazard rate for regional recurrence in women whose sentinel nodes are negative by H&E staining;
- To provide a mechanism for identifying women whose sentinel nodes contain metastases detected by H&E so that these women can be considered as candidates for ACOSOG Study Z0011.

Scheme:

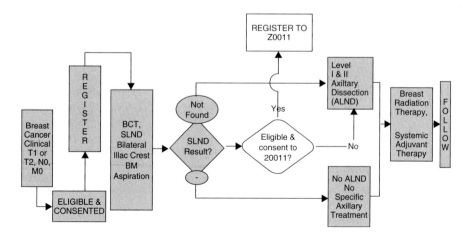

All patients enrolled in this study will be treated using *breast-conserving therapy (BCT)*. *BCT* consists of *segmental mastectomy* (lumpectomy), and *sentinel lymph node dissection* with the intent to treat with postoperative whole *breast radiation therapy* and, if clinically indicated, *systemic adjuvant therapy*. In addition, *bilateral anterior iliac crest bone marrow aspiration* will be performed prior to *BCT*.

When a sentinel node is NOT identified during the SLND, a level I and II axillary lymph node dissection (ALND) is performed. Patients who have no sentinel lymph node metastasis by H&E should not have an ALND. Patients with evidence of metastatic disease in the sentinel node may be eligible for registration and randomization to ACOSOG Z0011.

The results of disease-related assessments and treatment directed at breast cancer will be reported at 6, 12, 18, 24, 30 and 36 months following registration, and then yearly until death. Patients will be monitored for local and regional recurrence (especially recurrence in the ipsilateral axillary bed), contralateral breast primary tumors, distant recurrence, progression, and death. Special assessments for surgical side effects in the axillary bed and arms will be done on all patients.

Update:

Z0010 closed (met accural goal).

ACOSOG

Title: A randomized trial of axillary node dissection in women with clinical T1 or T2 N0 M0 breast cancer who have a positive sentinel node.
ACOSOG Z0011

Principal investigator: A.E. Giuliano
John Wayne Cancer Institute
2200 Santa Monica Boulevard, Suite 113
SANTA MONICA, CA 90404-2302
USA
Tel: +1 310 829 8089
Fax: +1 310 998 3995

Summary:
- Opened May 17, 1999
- Target accrual: 1900 eligible and evaluable patients

Objectives:

- To assess whether overall survival for patients randomized to Arm 2 (no immediate ALND) is equivalent to (or better) than that for patients assigned to Arm 1 (completion ALND);
- To quantify and compare the surgical morbidities associated with sentinel lymph node dissection (SLND) plus ALND versus SLND alone.

Scheme:

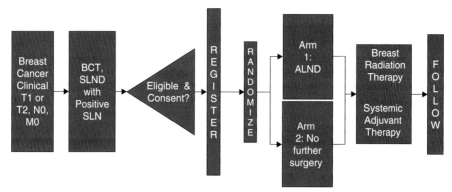

A patient will be eligible for this trial only if metastatic tumor is detected in the sentinel node by routine histopathology, either on frozen section, touch prep, or permanent section. The patient will be randomized to either Arm 1 or Arm 2, where the interventions associated with these Arms are as follows:

Arm 1: Axillary lymph node dissection (ALND), followed by adjuvant breast radiation therapy and, if indicated, adjuvant systemic therapy.

Arm 2: Breast radiation therapy and, if indicated, adjuvant systemic therapy only.

All patients, regardless of when they are randomized, and which arm they are assigned to, should be treated with whole breast radiation therapy and, if indicated, adjuvant systemic therapy. Special assessments for surgical side effects in the axillary bed and arms will be done within 30 days following the last study-related surgery, and at months 6, 12 and then yearly. The results of disease-related assessments and treatment directed at breast cancer will be reported at 6, 12, 18, 24, 30, and 36 months following registration, and then yearly until death or lost to follow-up. Patients will be monitored for local and regional recurrence (especially recurrence in the ipsilateral axillary bed), contralateral breast primary tumors, distant recurrence, progression, and death.

Update:

Accrual to date (11 July 2003): 587 patients.

CALGB

Title: Phase III double-blind, placebo-controlled, prospective randomized comparison of adjuvant therapy with tamoxifen vs tamoxifen and fenretinide in postmenopausal women with involved axillary lymph nodes and positive receptors.
INT-0151

Principal Investigator: M.A. Cobleigh
Rush-Presbyterian-St Luke's Medical Center
Professional Building, Suite 821
1725 West Harrison St.
CHICAGO, IL 60612-3863
USA
Tel: +1 312 942 3240
Fax: +1 312 942 3192
Email: mac@sispro.sis.rpslmc.edu

Summary:
- Opened in 1995
- Target accrual: 1500 patients

Objective:

To compare disease-free survival and overall survival of postmenopausal primary breast cancer patients with involved axillary nodes and positive estrogen or progesterone receptors who are treated with standard adjuvant tamoxifen vs tamoxifen and fenretinide.

Scheme: **Arm 1:** Tamoxifen (20 mg q am) × 5 yrs + placebo (4 capsules q pm) × 5 yrs
Arm 2: Tamoxifen (20 mg q am) × 5 yrs + fenretinide (4 capsules q pm) × 5 yrs

Update:

391 patients accrued through July 1999.

Title: Phase II study of trastuzumab (Herceptin) and gefitinib in patients with metastatic breast cancer that overexpresses HER2-neu.
E1100

Study Lead Organization: Eastern Cooperative Oncology Group
Carlos Arteaga, MD, Protocol chair
Tel: +615 936 1782; +1 800 811 8480

Scheme: Patients will receive gefitinib by mouth once a day for as long as benefit is shown. They will also receive an infusion of trastuzumab once a week for approximately 6 months followed by trastuzumab once every 3 weeks for as long as benefit is shown. Patients will be evaluated every 3 months for 2 years, every 6 months for 3 years, and once a year thereafter.

ECOG

Title: Phase III randomized study of paclitaxel with or without bevacizumab in patients with locally recurrent or metastatic breast cancer.
E2100

Study Lead Organization: Eastern Cooperative Oncology Group
Kathy Miller, MD, Protocol chair
Tel: +317 274 0920

Scheme: Patients will be randomly assigned to one of two groups. Patients in group one will receive an infusion of paclitaxel in weeks 1–3 and an infusion of bevacizumab in weeks 1 and 3. Patients in group two will receive paclitaxel alone as in group one. Treatment in both groups may be repeated every 4 weeks for up to 18 courses. Quality of life will be assessed periodically. Patients will be evaluated every 3 months for 2 years, every 6 months for 3 years, and once a year thereafter.

Title:

A phase III randomized study of doxorubicin / docetaxel vs doxorubicin / cyclophosphamide as adjuvant treatment for node-positive or high-risk node-negative breast cancer.
E2197

Principal Investigator:

L.J. Goldstein
Breast Evaluation Center
Fox Chase Cancer Center
7701 Burholme Ave #C307
PHILADELPHIA, PA 19111-2412
USA
Tel: +1 215 728 2689
Fax: +1 215 728 3639
Email: lj_goldstein@fccc.edu

Summary:

- Opened in 1998
- Target accrual: 2500 patients

Objectives:

- To determine whether doxorubicin / docetaxel (DD) will improve disease-free survival and overall survival when compared to doxorubicin / cyclophosphamide (DC) in patients with lymph node-positive (1–3 positive nodes) or high-risk lymph node-negative breast cancer;
- To compare the toxicity of DD to DC in this patient population.

Scheme:

Arm 1: DD
Arm 2: DC

For postmenopausal, ER+ and/or PR+ patients on both arms, followed by tamoxifen. This is recommended for premenopausal, ER+ and/or PR+ patients.

Update:

Trial closed to accrual 21 January 2000.

ECOG

Title: Phase II study of doxorubicin HCl liposome and docetaxel with or without trastuzumab (Herceptin) in women with metastatic breast cancer.
E3198

Study Lead Organization: Eastern Cooperative Oncology Group
Antonio C. Wolff, MD, Protocol chair
Tel: +410 614 4192

Scheme: Patients will be assigned to one of two treatment groups. Patients in group one will receive infusions of liposomal doxorubicin and docetaxel every 3 weeks for eight courses. They may then receive infusions of docetaxel alone either weekly or every 3 weeks for as long as benefit is shown. Patients in group two will receive an infusion of trastuzumab once a week, plus infusions of liposomal doxorubicin and docetaxel as in group one. They may then receive trastuzumab once a week followed by docetaxel either once a week or every 3 weeks for as long as benefit is shown. Patients will be evaluated every 3 months for 2 years, every 6 months for 3 years, and once a year thereafter.

Title: Local excision alone for selected patients with DCIS of the breast. E5194

Principal Investigator: L.L. Hughes
The Emory Clinic
Dept of Radiation Oncology
1365 Clifton Road
ATLANTA, GA 30322
USA
Tel: +1 404 778 4469
Fax: +1 404 778 4139

Summary:
- Opened in 1997
- Target accrual: 1176 patients

Objective:

To evaluate the 5- and 10-year actuarial local recurrence rate (in situ or invasive) after local excision alone for patients with favorable prognosis DCIS defined as: low or intermediate grade DCIS 2.5 cm or high grade DCIS 1 cm.

Scheme: All patients have breast-conserving surgery and are then followed with standardized clinical and mammographic follow-up care.

Update:

Trial closed to accrual 22 October 2002.

NSABP

Title: A three-arm randomized trial to compare adjuvant Adriamycin and cyclophosphamide followed by Taxotere (AC → T); Adriamycin and Taxotere (AT); Adriamycin, Taxotere, and cyclophosphamide (ATC) in breast cancer patients with positive axillary lymph nodes.
NSABP B-30

Principal Investigator: Norman Wolmark, MD
National Surgical Adjuvant Breast and Bowel Project
East Commons Professional Building
Four Allegheny Center, 5th Floor
PITTSBURGH, PA 15212-5234
USA

Summary:
- Opened March 15, 1999
- Target accrual: 5300 patients

Objectives:

- To compare the efficacy of adjuvant doxorubicin, cyclophosphamide, and docetaxel given concurrently vs adjuvant doxorubicin and cyclophosphamide followed by docetaxel in prolonging the overall survival and disease-free survival of breast cancer patients with positive axillary lymph nodes;
- To compare the efficacy of adjuvant doxorubicin and docetaxel vs regimens containing cyclophosphamide in these patients;
- To compare the toxicity of these three regimens in these patients;
- To compare the quality of life of the study patients;
- To compare the differences in amenorrhea in premenopausal women in each treatment arm and its relationship to symptoms, quality of life, and survival.

Scheme:
Arm I: Doxorubicin and cyclophosphamide followed by docetaxel
Arm II: Doxorubicin and docetaxel
Arm III: Doxorubicin, docetaxel, and cyclophosphamide

Tamoxifen will be given to all patients whose tumors are ER+ and/or PgR+. At the discretion of the investigator anastrozole may be given to postmenopausal patients as an alternative to tamoxifen.

Update:

3898 patients have been accrued through January 2003.

Title: A randomized trial comparing the safety and efficacy of Adriamycin and Cyclophosphamide followed by Taxol (AC → T) to that of Adriamycin and Cyclophosphamide followed by Taxol plus Herceptin (AC → T + H) in node-positive breast cancer patients who have tumors that overexpress HER2.
NSABP B-31

Principal Investigator: Norman Wolmark, MD
National Surgical Adjuvant Breast and Bowel Project
East Commons Professional Building
Four Allegheny Center, 5th Floor
PITTSBURGH, PA 15212-5234
USA

Summary:
- Opened February 21, 2000
- Target accrual: 2700 patients

Objectives:

- To compare the cardiotoxicity of doxorubicin and cyclophosphamide followed by paclitaxel with or without trastuzumab in patients with operable, node-positive breast cancer that overexpresses HER2;
- To compare the effect of these regimens, with or without tamoxifen, on prolonging overall survival and disease-free survival of these patients.

Scheme: Arm I: Doxorubicin and cyclophosphamide followed by paclitaxel
Arm II: Doxorubicin and cyclophosphamide followed by paclitaxel + trastuzumab

Update:

1241 patients have been accrued through January 2003.

NSABP

Title: A study to determine the correlation of cardiac function with patient characteristics and blood markers in women enrolled in NSABP B-31.1

Principal Investigator: Norman Wolmark, MD
National Surgical Adjuvant Breast and Bowel Project
East Commons Professional Building
Four Allegheny Center, 5th Floor
PITTSBURGH, PA 15212-5234
USA

Summary:
- Opened November 2001
- Target accrual: 220 patients

Objectives:

- To evaluate trastuzumab-associated abnormalities via echocardiographically obtained parameters indicative of diastolic dysfunction and correlate these abnormalities with baseline patient characteristics to help predict which patients are at greater risk of developing cardiac dysfunction when treated with doxorubicin and cyclophosphamide followed by paclitaxel with trastuzumab;
- To determine whether abnormal levels of brain natriuretic peptide, troponin-T, troponin-I, tumor necrosis factor-alpha, interleukin-1 beta, and interleukin-6 correlate with echocardiographic abnormalities that reflect myocardial damage in patients receiving doxorubicin and cyclophosphamide followed by paclitaxel with trastuzumab;
- To evaluate whether any of the blood markers can serve as early predictors of cardiac dysfunction in this adjuvant setting.

Scheme: Patients who enroll in this trial must also participate in NSABP B-31. All patients will undergo five echocardiograms and six blood collections over a period of 18 months, as well as have five patient visits where various patient characteristics, such as resting heart rate, blood pressure, and current medications, will be collected.

Update:

10 patients have been accrued through January 2003.

Title: A randomized phase III clinical trial to compare sentinel node resection to conventional axillary dissection in clinically node-negative breast cancer patients.
NSABP B-32

Principal Investigator: Norman Wolmark, MD
National Surgical Adjuvant Breast and Bowel Project
East Commons Professional Building
Four Allegheny Center, 5th Floor
PITTSBURGH, PA 15212-5234
USA

Summary:
- Opened May 17, 1999
- Target accrual: 5400 patients

Objectives:

- To compare the long-term control of regional disease by sentinel node resection alone vs sentinel node resection followed by conventional axillary dissection in women with breast cancer who are clinically node negative and pathologically sentinel node negative;
- To compare the morbidity and the effect of these two regimens on the overall and disease-free survival of these patients;
- To compare the prognostic value of these two regimens in patients who are sentinel node negative or sentinel node positive by pathology;
- To determine in patients who are sentinel node negative by pathology if a more detailed pathology investigation of sentinel nodes can identify a group of patients with a potentially increased risk of systemic recurrence;
- To determine whether self-assessed symptoms and activity limitations will be more severe in Group 1 than Group 2;
- To determine whether self-assessed symptoms and activity limitations after breast cancer surgery are more severe in women whose surgery was on the dominant side, compared with women whose surgery was on the non-dominant side;
- To determine the affect of arm edema, range of motion, and sensory neuropathy on self-assessed measures of daily functioning, symptoms, and overall quality of life.

Scheme:
Arm I: Sentinel node resection followed by immediate conventional axillary node dissection.

Arm II: Sentinel node biopsy with intraoperative node exam; if sentinel node is negative, no further surgery; if sentinel node is positive, a conventional axillary node dissection will be performed immediately.

Update:

4435 patients have been accrued through January 2003.

NSABP

Title: A randomized, placebo-controlled, double-blind trial evaluating the effect of exemestane in clinical stage T_{1-3} N_{0-1} M_0 postmenopausal breast cancer patients completing at least five years of tamoxifen therapy.
NSABP B-33

Principal Investigator: Norman Wolmark, MD
National Surgical Adjuvant Breast and Bowel Project
East Commons Professional Building
Four Allegheny Center, 5th Floor
PITTSBURGH, PA 15212-5234
USA

Summary:
- Opened May 2001
- Target accrual: 3000 patients

Objectives:

- To determine whether the administration of 5 years of exemestane following 5 years of tamoxifen therapy is more effective than 5 years of tamoxifen alone in prolonging disease free survival, overall survival, and time to treatment failure in postmenopausal patients with resected estrogen receptor-positive and/or progesterone receptor-positive breast cancer;
- To evaluate the effect of tamoxifen withdrawal on bone;
- To evaluate the effect of exemestane on bone after tamoxifen withdrawal.

Scheme:
Arm I: Exemestane
Arm II: Placebo

Update:

866 patients have been accrued through January 2003.

Title:	A clinical trial comparing adjuvant clodronate therapy vs placebo in early-stage breast cancer patients receiving systemic chemotherapy and/or tamoxifen or no therapy. NSABP B-34
Principal Investigator:	Norman Wolmark, MD National Surgical Adjuvant Breast and Bowel Project East Commons Professional Building Four Allegheny Center, 5th Floor PITTSBURGH, PA 15212-5234 USA
Summary:	• Opened December 1, 2000 • Target accrual: 3200 patients

Objectives:

- To determine whether clodronate administered for 3 years either alone or in addition to adjuvant chemotherapy and/or hormonal therapy, in patients with early-stage breast cancer will improve disease-free survival, overall survival, and relapse free survival;
- To determine whether clodronate will reduce the incidence of skeletal metastases, non-skeletal metastases, and skeletal morbidity;
- To investigate the relevance of serum markers of bone turnover as a prognostic factor for the development of bone metastasis.

Scheme: **Arm I:** Clodronate
 Arm II: Placebo

Update:

1959 patients have been accrued through January 2003.

NSABP

Title: A clinical trial comparing anastrozole with tamoxifen in postmenopausal patients with ductal carcinoma in situ (DCIS) undergoing lumpectomy with radiation therapy. NSABP B-35

Principal Investigator: Norman Wolmark, MD
National Surgical Adjuvant Breast and Bowel Project
East Commons Professional Building
Four Allegheny Center, 5th Floor
PITTSBURGH, PA 15212-5234
USA

Summary:
- Opened January 2003
- Target accrual: 3000 patients

Objectives:

- To compare the value of 1 mg/day of anastrozole to 20 mg/day of tamoxifen, each given for 5 years, in preventing the subsequent occurrence of breast cancer (local, regional and distant recurrences, and contralateral breast cancer) following lumpectomy with radiation therapy in postmenopausal women with ductal carcinoma in situ (DCIS);
- To compare the quality of life of the patients between the two arms;
- To compare the two arms in terms of osteoporotic fractures;
- To compare the two arms in terms of future malignancies;
- To compare the two arms in terms of disease free survival and overall survival.

Scheme: **Arm I:** Tamoxifen + placebo + Breast Radiation Therapy
Arm II: Anastrozole + placebo + Breast Radiation Therapy

Update:

1 patient has been accrued as of February 2003.

Title: Study of Tamoxifen and Raloxifene for the Prevention of Breast Cancer. STAR

Co-ordinator: Norman Wolmark, MD
National Surgical Adjuvant Breast and Bowel Project
East Commons Professional Building
Four Allegheny Center, 5th Floor
PITTSBURGH, PA 15212-5234
USA

Summary:

- Target accrual: 19,000 women

Objective:

To determine whether raloxifene is more or less effective than tamoxifen in significantly reducing the incidence rate of invasive breast cancer in postmenopausal women.

Inclusion:

- Postmenopausal women at increased risk for developing invasive breast cancer.
- Defined as histologically confirmed lobular carcinoma in situ treated by local excision only or at least 1.66% probability of invasive breast cancer within 5 years using Breast Cancer Risk Assessment Profile.
- Women 35 years of age and over.

Exclusion:

- Evidence of malignant disease on physical exam within 180 days, or mammogram within past year.
- Prophylactic mastectomy.
- Prior history of invasive cancer or intraductal carcinoma in situ.
- No other prior malignancy within past 5 years except basal cell or squamous cell carcinoma of the skin and carcinoma in situ of the cervix.
- Contraindications to use of tamoxifen or raloxifene.

Follow Up:

- Clinical and mammography.
- Quality of life is assessed at baseline every 6 months until 60 months.
- Patients are followed annually after 5 years.

Primary End Points:

- Breast Cancer

Scheme: **Arm I**: Patients receive oral tamoxifen plus placebo daily for 5 years.
  Arm II: Patients receive oral raloxifene plus placebo daily for 5 years.

Update:

15,285 participants accrued through January 2003.

References:

Vogel VG, Costantino JP, Wickerham DL et al. The Study of Tamoxifen and Raloxifene: Preliminary Enrollment Data from a Randomized Breast Cancer Risk Reduction Trial. *Clin Breast Cancer* 3:153–159, 2002.

Title:	Phase III trial of observation +/− tamoxifen vs RT +/− tamoxifen for good risk duct carcinoma in situ *(DCIS)* of the female breast. RTOG 9804

Principal Investigator:

Beryl McCormick, MD
Memorial Sloan-Kettering Cancer Center
1275 York Avenue, Room H208
NEW YORK, NY 10021
USA
Tel: +1 (212) 639 6828
Fax: +1 (212) 639 8876
Email: mccormib@mskcc.org

Summary:

- Opened in December 1999
- Target accrual: 1790 patients

Objectives:

- To compare the efficacy of tamoxifen with or without whole breast radiation, in decreasing or delaying the appearance of local failure, both invasive and in situ, and preventing the need for mastectomy in women with ductal carcinoma in situ (DCIS) of the breast;
- To compare distant disease-free survival of these patients in these treatment arms.

Scheme:

Patients with low or intermediate grade DCIS following surgery are eligible. Patients are randomized to: No Radiation therapy (observation) or Radiation therapy (16–28 fractions of radiotherapy for total dose of 42.5–50.4Gy).

Use of tamoxifen is optional on both arms. Prior to randomization, the physician must specify if patient will be given tamoxifen or not. Tamoxifen is given 20 mg daily for 5 years.

(See RTOG website – see contact details)

Update:

265 patients accrued through February 2003.